ARRHYTHMIA INTERPRETATION

A WORKBOOK FOR NURSES

ARRHYTHMIA
INTERPRETATION
A WORKBOOK FOR NURSES

Joanne Noone, RN, MSN, CEN, CCRN
Medical-Surgical Nursing Instructor
Kauai Community College
Lihue, Hawaii

Springhouse Corporation
Springhouse, Pennsylvania

Staff

Executive Director, Editorial
Stanley Loeb

Director of Trade and Textbooks
Minnie B. Rose, RN, BSN, MEd

Art Director
John Hubbard

Editors
David Moreau, Karen Zimmermann

Clinical Consultants
Maryann Foley, RN, BSN; Cindy Tryniszewski, RN, MSN, CS

Drug Information Editor
George J. Blake, RPh, MS

Copy Editors
Mary Hohenhaus Hardy, Pamela Wingrod

Design
Stephanie Peters (associate art director), Mary Stangl (book designer)

Manufacturing
Deborah Meiris (manager), T.A. Landis

Library of Congress Cataloging – in – Publication Data

Noone, Joanne, 1956–
    Arrhythmia interpretation: a workbook for nurses / Joanne Noone.
    p.   cm.
    Includes bibliographical references and index.
    1. Arrhythmia–Nursing. I.Title.
    [DNLM: 1. Arrhythmia–diagnosis–nurses' instruction.
2. Arrhythmia–nursing.   WG 330 N817a]
RC685.A65N66 1992   616.1'2807547'024613–dc20   DNLM/DLC
ISBN 0–87434–402–6   91–5237 CIP

Contents

Acknowledgments

I want to express my gratitude to Beatrice Fulcher, RN, who first taught me the art of ECG interpretation. From time to time when teaching my classes, I hear myself repeating her maxims on arrhythmia interpretation and treatment.

Over the years, many other nurses have shared pearls of wisdom with me as I have tried to decipher a difficult rhythm or interpret a 12-lead ECG during a crisis. To all those nurses, I extend my heartfelt thanks.

I also must recognize Laura Gasparis Vonfrolio, the driving force in motivating me to write this book and the first person to acknowledge the writer in me. I am fortunate to have her as a mentor.

Last, I extend thanks to Maryann Foley, my clinical editor, for her advice and support in making this book a reality.

Dedication
To James and Harry, whose anticipated arrival hastened the completion of this book

Preface

This book is for the ever-increasing number of practicing nurses — those working in medical-surgical units, critical care units, emergency departments, operating rooms, postanesthesia care units, outpatient clinics, and various community settings — who are responsible for interpreting the client's heart rhythm as a part of their job requirement. My awareness of the need for nurses to attain this skill was first heightened by an experience I had years ago. Soon after graduating from nursing school, I worked in a medical neurology unit. Caring for clients on cardiac monitors was rare then, but one evening I was assigned to care for a woman with an acute cerebrovascular accident whose medication orders included a lidocaine drip for PVCs. After looking up lidocaine in the *Physicians' Desk Reference,* I asked the assignment nurse, "What are PVCs?" He drew one out for me, cautioning me to call the physician if more than six PVCs occurred in 1 minute. Not until a year later, after I began working in a coronary care unit, did I come to realize that my nursing school training had left me ill-prepared to care for such clients.

A few years ago, I returned to the medical-surgical nursing arena, this time as a nursing instructor. Noting the increase in client acuity and the need for medical-surgical nurses to have a working knowledge of arrhythmia interpretation, I became committed to teaching my students this information in an elective course, to prepare them to work in real clinical settings. In searching for an appropriate text, I discovered that most ECG books fall into one of three categories: some combine basic and advanced interpretation, overwhelming the newcomer; some are written by and for physicians, thus failing to meet the needs of a nursing audience; and some discuss the arrhythmia but not the treatment, leaving the learner to practice in a void.

Arrhythmia Interpretation: A Workbook for Nurses fills that void; in clear, concise language, it teaches the nurse how to interpret arrhythmias *and* how to respond appropriately.

Chapter 1 reviews basic principles of cardiac anatomy, physiology, and electrophysiology; topics include the heart's major structures and functions, the cardiac conduction system, and depolarization and repolarization, among others.

Chapter 2 describes the electrocardiogram, the 12-lead ECG, components of the ECG complex, and heart rate measurement; additionally, the chapter provides a systematic approach to ECG interpretation that should benefit all nurses beginning to learn about cardiac arrhythmias.

Chapters 3 to 7 focus on interpretation of the major arrhythmias: sinus bradycardia, sinus tachycardia, sinus arrhythmia, sinus arrest and exit block, premature atrial contraction, paroxysmal and nonparoxysmal atrial tachycardia, atrial flutter, atrial fibrillation, wandering atrial pacemaker, multifocal atrial tachycardia, premature junctional contraction, junctional rhythm, accelerated junctional rhythm, junctional tachycardia, premature ventricular contraction, ventricular tachycardia, ventricular fibrillation, idioventricular rhythm, accelerated idioventricular rhythm, asystole, and first-, second-, and third-degree AV blocks.

Chapter 8 describes the indications for and common complications of temporary and permanent pacemakers and provides a systematic approach to assessing properly paced rhythms.

To enhance learning, this workbook uses a step-by-step approach to arrhythmia interpretation. First, for each rhythm presented, the text describes ECG characteristics, effects on the client, standard treatments, and implications for the nurse. Next, to help the reader assess knowledge gained, practice examples appear after the discussion of each arrhythmia (correct answers appear later in the chapter). Finally, self-tests at the end of each chapter provide additional practice opportunities (correct answers appear in Appendix A). Numerous illustrations and tables throughout the text clarify key concepts, and 20 post-tests with correct answers (Appendix B) provide still further opportunities for practice and review. To assist the reader in planning, Appendix C offers nursing care plans for selected arrhythmias, including pertinent nursing diagnoses, expected outcomes, and nursing interventions. The workbook concludes with selected references for additional reading and a handy index for locating important topics quickly.

Arrhythmia Interpretation: A Workbook for Nurses is an ideal resource for practicing nurses who are new to ECG interpretation or who want a refresher; its design enables self-learners to proceed at their own pace. As an adjunct to classroom learning, the book will give nursing school students the opportunity to sharpen their interpretation skills before graduation so they will be better prepared to meet their responsibilities afterward. With practice and determination, the diligent reader will reaffirm this book's ultimate purpose — to promote competent nursing care for all clients.

Cardiac Anatomy, Physiology, and Electrophysiology

To understand how arrhythmias are formed and to recognize their implications for the client, the nurse must have a working knowledge of cardiac anatomy, physiology, and electrophysiology. This chapter can provide such a knowledge base. It describes the heart's major structures and functions, reviews the cardiac conduction system and coronary circulation, and explains such important concepts as autonomic innervation, the properties of cardiac cells, depolarization and repolarization, and the action potential. The chapter concludes by examining the underlying causes and clinical relevance of arrhythmias.

LOCATION OF THE HEART

The heart is located behind the sternum, in the mediastinal cavity formed between the right and left lungs. It lies within a pericardial sac, and its only attachment to the thorax is through the great vessels — aorta, inferior and superior venae cavae, pulmonary arteries, and pulmonary veins.

Locating the heart in the thorax

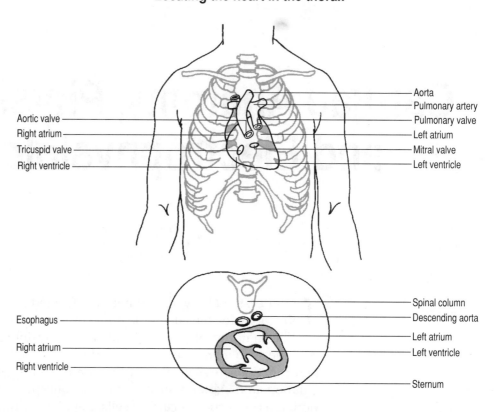

The heart's position is oblique, with the right ventricle situated toward the front (anteriorly) of the chest and the left ventricle to the side (laterally). The base of the cone-shaped heart lies to the right and in a posterior position, beneath the second rib. The apex of the heart lies to the left in an anterior position, at the fifth intercostal space, midclavicular line. There, the heart's apex can be palpated. This clinical finding is called the point of maximal impulse.

LAYERS OF THE HEART

The three layers of the heart are the pericardium, the myocardium, and the endocardium.

Layers of the heart

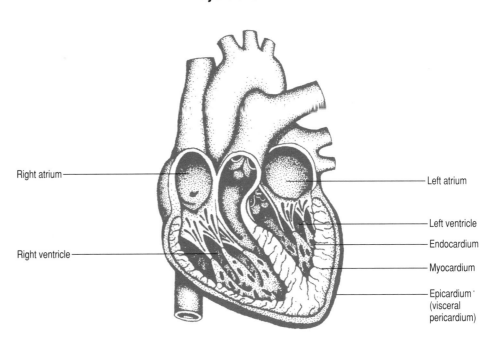

Right atrium —

Right ventricle —

— Left atrium

— Left ventricle

— Endocardium

— Myocardium

— Epicardium · (visceral pericardium)

The pericardium is the outermost lining of the heart and consists of two layers — the parietal (outer) pericardium and the visceral (inner) pericardium, also called the epicardium. The inner and outer layers are separated by approximately 10 ml of serous fluid, which acts as a lubricant. The pericardium has three functions: holding the heart in place within the mediastinum, reducing friction over the heart's moving surface, and protecting the heart from bacterial or neoplastic invasion.

The middle and thickest layer of the heart, the myocardium, contains the contractile myocardial fibers, as well as the conduction system and blood supply. The chambers under highest pressure have the thickest musculature. Thus, ventricular tissue is thicker than atrial tissue because the ventricles must achieve higher pressures to eject blood. The left ventricle has the thickest musculature because it must eject blood against the arterial blood pressure in the aorta, the vessel under the highest pressure.

The endocardium is a lining of endothelial tissue within the heart and valves. Blood is provided to the heart's valves and internal lining through the intimal (inner) layer of blood vessels connected to the endocardium.

HEART CHAMBERS

The heart consists of four chambers — the right atrium, right ventricle, left atrium, and left ventricle.

Heart chambers

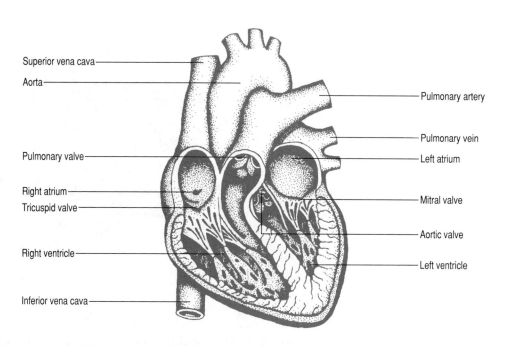

The right atrium receives deoxygenated blood from the superior and inferior venae cavae and sends it to the right ventricle through the tricuspid valve. The right ventricle ejects the blood into the pulmonary arteries via the pulmonary valve. The pulmonary arteries take the blood to the lungs, where oxygen and carbon dioxide are exchanged. Pulmonary veins take the newly oxygenated blood to the left atrium, which acts as a conduit, sending blood though the mitral valve to the left ventricle. From the left ventricle, the blood is ejected through the aortic valve into the aorta, the coronary arteries, and the systemic circulation.

The two atria and the right ventricle are normally low-pressure chambers that pump against low resistance. However, valvular, pulmonary, or left-ventricular disease, as well as systemic hypertension, can increase the resistance against which these chambers pump, thereby increasing their pressure. The left ventricle is normally a high-pressure chamber that must exceed the arterial pressure to eject its contents.

The atria contract simultaneously, preceding ventricular contraction. During diastole (the relaxation phase of the cardiac cycle), the atria function as passive conduits, allowing blood to flow through them into the ventricles. Just before ventricular systole (the contraction phase of the cardiac cycle), the atria contract, pumping the rest of their contents into the ventricles, which then simultaneously eject blood into the pulmonary and systemic circulations. The atrial contraction, called *atrial kick*, accounts for 10% to 30% of the cardiac output, the amount of blood ejected from the left ventricle. Atrial kick is lost in arrhythmias that alter synchronous contraction between the atria and the ventricles. Such arrhythmias may reduce cardiac output in clients with minimal cardiac reserve, such as those with an enlarged heart from hypertension or borderline congestive heart failure.

HEART VALVES

Four valves in the heart prevent blood from flowing backward — the tricuspid valve, pulmonary valve, mitral valve, and aortic valve.

The tricuspid and mitral valves are called atrioventricular (AV) valves because of their location; the tricuspid valve separates the right atrium from the right ventricle, and the mitral valve separates the left atrium from the left ventricle. During diastole, these valves open to allow blood to flow from the atria to the ventricles; they close during systole to prevent blood from flowing back into the atria during contraction. The AV valves are attached to papillary muscles by thin, fibrous threads called chordae tendineae. Contraction of the papillary muscles keeps the valves closed during systole.

The pulmonary and aortic valves are called semilunar valves because of their shape: they consist of three half-moon cusps. These valves sit at the origin of the pulmonary artery and aorta, respectively. During systole, increased pressure in the ventricles opens these valves so that blood can be ejected into the pulmonary and systemic circulation. After systole, in-

Heart valves and muscles

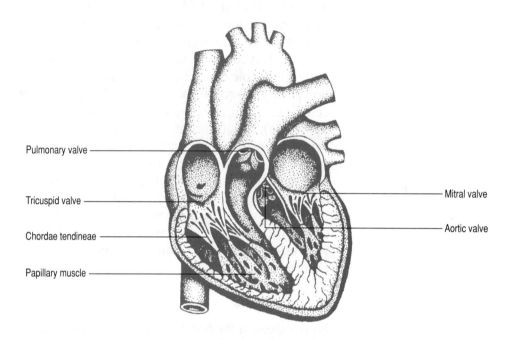

creased pressure in the arteries closes the valves so that the ventricles can fill with blood during diastole.

CONDUCTION SYSTEM

The heart contains specialized conductive tissue that can spontaneously generate and conduct an electrical impulse, which makes the cardiac muscle contract. Components of the conduction system are the sinoatrial (SA) node, the internodal and interatrial fibers, the AV node, the bundle of His, the bundle branches, and the Purkinje fibers.

All these components have the property of conductivity, or the ability to conduct electrical impulses. However, under normal conditions, only the SA node, the AV junction (the AV node and the bundle of His), and the Purkinje fibers have the property of automaticity, or the ability to generate an impulse spontaneously.

The SA node is considered the heart's pacemaker. Located high in the right atrium, it spontaneously fires at a rate of 60 to 100 beats/minute. The impulse generated by the SA node is conducted to the left atrium by Bachmann's bundle and to the AV node by the internodal tracts.

Conduction system

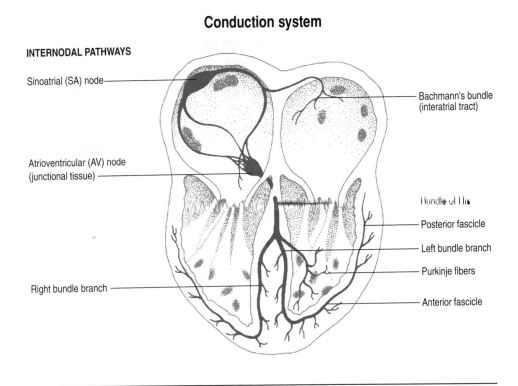

INTERNODAL PATHWAYS

Sinoatrial (SA) node

Atrioventricular (AV) node
(junctional tissue)

Right bundle branch

Bachmann's bundle
(interatrial tract)

Bundle of His

Posterior fascicle

Left bundle branch

Purkinje fibers

Anterior fascicle

The AV node sits low in the right atrium, near the tricuspid valve. It delays the SA node's impulse for 0.04 second to allow for atrial contraction, then sends the impulse to the ventricles via the bundle of His. The AV junction, which can serve as a back-up pacemaker, has an inherent rate of 40 to 60 beats/minute.

The bundle of His conducts the impulse to the right and left bundle branches. The right bundle branch innervates the right ventricle, and the left bundle branch divides into two fascicles, or bundles, to supply the larger left ventricle. These two bundles are called the left anterior fascicle and the left posterior fascicle. The impulse then travels to the Purkinje fibers, a network that infiltrates the ventricular myocardium. These fibers have an inherent pacemaker ability of 20 to 40 beats/minute.

CORONARY CIRCULATION

The heart is supplied with blood, mostly during diastole, by the right and left coronary arteries, which branch off the aorta.

Cardiac blood supply

These two views show the coronary arteries that supply the heart with blood and the main cardiac veins that drain it.

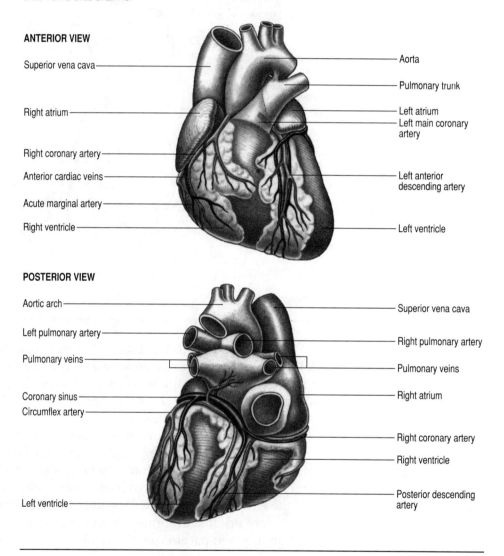

ANTERIOR VIEW

Superior vena cava

Right atrium

Right coronary artery

Anterior cardiac veins

Acute marginal artery

Right ventricle

Aorta

Pulmonary trunk

Left atrium

Left main coronary artery

Left anterior descending artery

Left ventricle

POSTERIOR VIEW

Aortic arch

Left pulmonary artery

Pulmonary veins

Coronary sinus

Circumflex artery

Left ventricle

Superior vena cava

Right pulmonary artery

Pulmonary veins

Right atrium

Right coronary artery

Right ventricle

Posterior descending artery

The right coronary artery supplies blood to the following heart structures:
- SA node in about 50% of the population
- AV node in about 90% of the population
- right atrium and right ventricle
- inferior wall of the left ventricle
- posterior wall in about 90% of the population.

The left coronary artery divides into the left anterior descending and the left circumflex arteries. The left anterior descending artery supplies blood to these heart structures:
• anterior surface of the left ventricle
• interventricular septum
• bundle of His
• right bundle branch
• left anterior fascicle.

The left circumflex artery supplies blood to these heart structures:
• lateral wall of the left ventricle
• left atrium
• SA node in about 50% of the population
• AV node in about 10% of the population
• posterior wall in about 10% of the population
• left posterior fascicle.

Venous blood flows through the coronary sinus, located posteriorly between the atria and the ventricles. The coronary sinus and its tributaries, the anterior cardiac veins and the thebesian veins, all drain into the right atrium.

AUTONOMIC INNERVATION

The heart is innervated by the sympathetic and parasympathetic nervous systems.

The sympathetic nervous system stimulates the heart and blood vessels via branches of the cervical and thoracic nerves. It also stimulates the heart through the effects of circulating catecholamines — norepinephrine and epinephrine. The actions of the sympathetic nervous system are categorized according to the different responses produced in innervated organs. These responses are classified as alpha, beta 1, or beta 2. To understand the effects of these responses on the heart and blood vessels, see *Cardiovascular response to sympathetic nervous system stimulation*.

Cardiovascular response to sympathetic nervous system stimulation

Receptor	Organ	Response
Alpha	Vascular smooth muscle	Arterial and venous vasoconstriction
Beta-1	Heart	Increased heart rate, AV conduction, and contractility; enhanced automaticity
Beta-2	None	None

Autonomic cardiac innervation

This diagram suggests how the sympathetic and parasympathetic nervous systems innervate the heart.

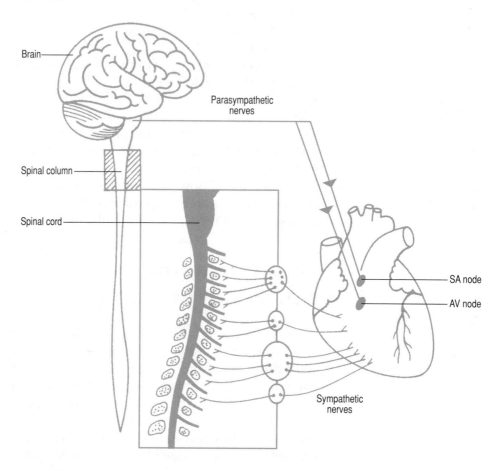

The vagus nerve, a cranial nerve with parasympathetic properties, decreases heart rate and slows impulse transmission through the AV node and the ventricular conduction system. Specialized nerve tissue, called baroreceptors, in the internal carotid arteries and the aorta are stimulated when stretched, such as occurs in hypertension. These receptors activate the vagus nerve to decrease heart rate and AV conduction. Baroreceptors in the carotid arteries can be mechanically stimulated as a therapeutic intervention to slow the heart rate or AV conduction. This is known as carotid sinus massage.

PROPERTIES OF CARDIAC CELLS

Cardiac cells have four different electrophysiologic properties — automaticity, excitability, conductivity, and contractility.

Specialized cells in the conduction system — specifically, the SA node, AV junction, and Purkinje fibers — have the property of automaticity (the ability to initiate an electrical impulse spontaneously). Because the SA node has the highest inherent impulse rate, it is the dominant pacemaker of the heart. Other cardiac cells not part of the conductive tissue may have their automaticity enhanced by certain conditions, such as hypoxia.

All cardiac cells have the properties of excitability (the ability to respond to an electrical impulse), conductivity (the ability to transmit the impulse to another cardiac cell), and contractility (the ability to contract after receiving a stimulus).

DEPOLARIZATION AND REPOLARIZATION

Depolarization and repolarization describe the changes that occur in the heart when an impulse forms and spreads throughout muscle tissue.

Understanding the depolarization–repolarization cycle

The depolarization-repolarization cycle, which produces the heart's electrical activity, consists of the following phases:

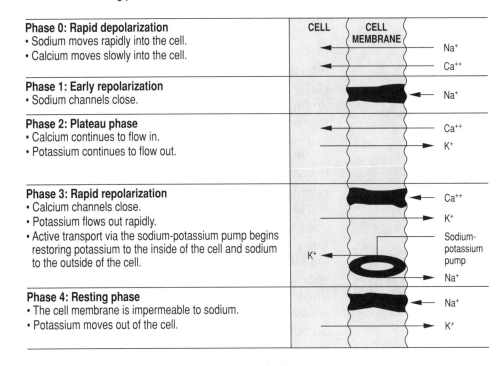

Phase 0: Rapid depolarization
- Sodium moves rapidly into the cell.
- Calcium moves slowly into the cell.

Phase 1: Early repolarization
- Sodium channels close.

Phase 2: Plateau phase
- Calcium continues to flow in.
- Potassium continues to flow out.

Phase 3: Rapid repolarization
- Calcium channels close.
- Potassium flows out rapidly.
- Active transport via the sodium-potassium pump begins restoring potassium to the inside of the cell and sodium to the outside of the cell.

Phase 4: Resting phase
- The cell membrane is impermeable to sodium.
- Potassium moves out of the cell.

During diastole, the resting heart is *polarized*, meaning that the inside of the cardiac cell is more negatively charged than the outside. Depolarization changes the electrical current inside the cell, whether the impulse is spontaneously generated or received by the cell.

The inside of the cell now becomes positively charged. Cardiac contraction occurs during depolarization. Repolarization occurs as the inside of the cardiac cell returns to its normal (negatively charged) state. Depolarization and repolarization occur in a five-phase cycle known as the action potential.

ACTION POTENTIAL

The action potential describes the changes in intracardiac voltage that lead to impulse formation and conduction and, ultimately, to cardiac contraction.

Before an impulse arrives, the inside of a cardiac cell is more negatively charged than the outside, measuring about –90 mV. This is called the resting membrane potential.

Phase 0 of the action potential is initiated when the cell receives an impulse. During this phase, sodium freely enters the cell, making it more positive, up to +20 to +30 mV. Phase 0 corresponds to depolarization and the onset of cardiac contraction. After this phase, the cell wall becomes impermeable to sodium.

Phase 1 is marked by early rapid repolarization. The inside of the cell during this phase measures about 0 mV.

Phase 2, the plateau phase, is a period of slow repolarization. During this phase, the cell remains positively charged from an influx of calcium, which is used for cardiac contraction. Unlike skeletal muscle, cardiac muscle has the property of a plateau phase, allowing cardiac fibers to contract and relax. During phases 1 and 2, the cardiac cell is said to be in its absolute refractory period. A stimulus, no matter how strong, will not excite a cardiac cell during this time.

Phase 3, the repolarization phase, occurs as the cell returns to its negative state from an outflow of potassium. During phase 3, the cell is in its relative refractory period; a very strong stimulus can depolarize a cardiac cell at this time.

Phase 4, which corresponds to diastole, is the resting phase of the action potential. The heart is polarized during this phase. The cardiac cell wall is impermeable to sodium, but potassium can leave freely in response to extracellular conditions to maintain the cell's negativity. (For an illustration of these concepts, see *Myocardial action potential curve*.)

Why do some cells have the property of automaticity while others do not? All cells, whether automatic or not, usually do not become permeable to sodium until the intracardiac voltage reaches –60 mV. This voltage, called the threshold potential, signifies the onset of depolarization

Myocardial action potential curve

and the influx of sodium. Cells with the property of automaticity have an unstable phase 4, meaning that the resting state of this type of cell is usually about –60 mV, or the point at which sodium normally begins to enter the cell. Therefore, these cells are more likely to initiate an action potential spontaneously.

CAUSES OF ARRHYTHMIAS

Arrhythmias can be caused by enhanced automaticity, reentry, escape beats, or conduction disturbances (see *How arrhythmias develop,* page 14).

In enhanced automaticity, cardiac cells without the property of automaticity begin to fire automatically. These impulses are referred to as *ectopic* rhythms, because they are initiated outside the normal conduction system. Enhanced automaticity of nonautomatic cardiac cells can be caused by administration of catecholamines or atropine sulfate, hypoxia, acidosis, alkalosis, hypokalemia, hypocalcemia, or digoxin toxicity. Under these conditions, cardiac cells may begin to have unstable phase 4 resting potentials and may become permeable to sodium, initiating depolarization.

In reentry, an impulse returns to stimulate previously depolarized tissue. When conducted slowly, the impulse either travels sluggishly through the myocardial tissue or is completely blocked. This situation can cause the tissues to have different refractory periods. The impulse usually dies out in the Purkinje fibers because all the tissue around these fibers is absolutely refractory; that is, it cannot respond to any stimulus. However, if an area becomes relatively refractory when it should be absolutely refractory, the impulse can return to the electrical conduction pathway, producing a premature beat or a short period of sustained tachyarrhythmias. Ischemia, electrolyte disturbances, and some antiarrhythmic drugs can cause reentry by slowing or blocking conduction.

Escape beats occur when the heart's pacemakers fail to initiate depolarization. Originating in the AV junction or the ventricles, escape beats are compensatory mechanisms to maintain cardiac output. Failure of the dominant pacemaker must be treated, not the escape beat.

How arrhythmias develop

Cause	Mechanism	Associated arrhythmias
Enhanced automaticity	Cells lose stability in phase 4	• Wandering atrial pacemaker • Multifocal atrial tachycardia • Atrial fibrillation • Atrial flutter • Premature atrial, junctional, or ventricular contractions • Supraventricular tachycardia • Accelerated junctional rhythm • Junctional tachycardia • Accelerated idioventricular rhythm • Ventricular tachycardia • Ventricular fibrillation
Reentry	Impulse reenters previously depolarized tissue	• Premature atrial, junctional, or ventricular contractions • Paroxysmal supraventricular tachycardia • Ventricular tachycardia • Ventricular fibrillation
Escape beats	Dominant pacemaker fails to initiate depolarization	• Junctional rhythm • Idioventricular rhythm • Accelerated idioventricular rhythm
Conduction disturbance	Conduction system is impaired	• Sinus bradycardia • Sinus arrest • Sinus exit block • First-degree AV block • Second-degree AV block • Third-degree AV block • Asystole

Conduction disturbances may be temporary or permanent. The conduction system can be impaired or injured by cardiac surgery, trauma, myocardial ischemia or infarction, congenital heart disease, infectious diseases (such as syphilis), electrolyte disturbances, and drug toxicity.

CHAPTER 2

Electrocardiography

Because of its life-saving potential, arrhythmia interpretation is one of the most important skills that nurses can develop — and one of the most challenging to master. For those beginning to learn about cardiac arrhythmias, this chapter provides an introduction to the principles of electrocardiography, which lays the foundation for arrhythmia interpretation. The text first explains the different components of the electrocardiogram (ECG) complex and then demonstrates how to measure heart rates and intervals using ECG strips. Rounding out the discussion is a systematic approach to arrhythmia interpretation that provides a consistent and effective method of analysis for the nurse new to ECG interpretation.

ELECTROCARDIOGRAM

An ECG records electrical activity within the heart through electrodes placed at certain points on the client's skin. The electrodes, which can be disks, metal plates, or suction cups, are attached by cables to the ECG machine.

The ECG aids in the diagnosis of many cardiac and noncardiac conditions, including myocardial ischemia and infarction; cardiac conduction disturbances; arrhythmias; cardiac chamber enlargement; electrolyte disturbances, especially of potassium and calcium; effects of drugs, such as digoxin; and pulmonary hypertension, pulmonary embolism, and pericarditis. Serial ECGs, which are taken over time, document changes in the heart's electrical activity. Interpreting these changes provides vital information about the client's condition.

For an accurate and complete client profile, the ECG record must be interpreted in conjunction with the client's history and with clinical information obtained from physical assessment and diagnostic tests.

12–LEAD ECG

Electrical currents flow from the heart simultaneously in many different directions. For this reason, the heart's electrical activity should be seen from several viewpoints, which can be done using a 12-lead ECG. Each lead graphically represents a distinct area of the heart; the 12 leads together provide a complete picture of the heart's electrical activity.

Six of the 12 leads are called limb leads, because they detect electrical current emanating from the heart through electrodes placed on the client's limbs. The six limb leads — designated I, II, III, aV_R, aV_L, and aV_F — record electrical activity in the heart's frontal plane.

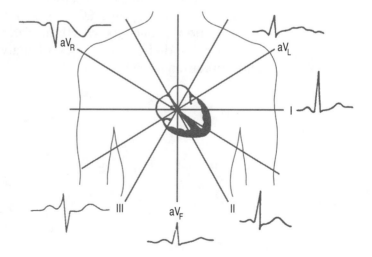

Leads I, II, and III are bipolar leads; they record electrical potentials (activity) between two electrodes, one positive and one negative. The positive electrode is always the recording electrode. In lead I, the right arm is negative, and the left arm is positive.

Lead I provides information about the left, or lateral, side of the heart. In lead II, the right arm is negative, and the left leg is positive. In lead III, the left arm is negative, and the left leg is positive. Leads II and III provide information about the inferior wall of the heart. Lead II is the conventional monitoring lead because P waves are upright and clearly visible in this lead.

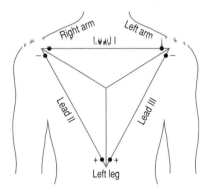

aV$_R$ (augmented vector right), aV$_L$ (augmented vector left), and aV$_F$ (augmented vector foot) are unipolar leads. With unipolar leads, a designated limb is the positive recording electrode in relation to the center of the heart, which is neutral.

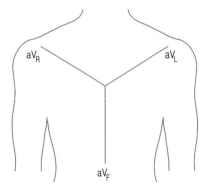

The right arm is the recording electrode for aV_R, the left arm for aV_L, and the left leg for aV_F. The ECG machine augments these leads by 50% because they initially produce small ECG complexes. aV_R provides information about electrical activity flowing to the right, aV_L about electrical activity flowing to the left, and aV_F about electrical activity flowing downward. Because little electrical current flows right, aV_R usually is not a useful lead for assessing a client's condition. aV_L provides data on activity in the lateral wall of the left ventricle, whereas aV_F provides data on activity in the inferior wall of the left ventricle.

The other six leads, called precordial leads, are placed on the chest wall. These leads are unipolar; the positive recording electrode is the lead that is moved about on the chest.

Precordial electrode placement

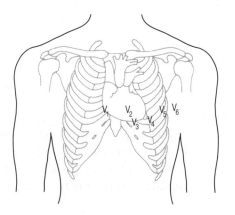

Lead	Positive electrode	Negative electrode
V_1	Fourth intercostal space at right border of sternum	Average potential of the three limbs: right arm, left arm, left leg
V_2	Fourth intercostal space at left border of sternum	
V_3	Approximately halfway between V_2 and V_4	
V_4	Fifth intercostal space at midclavicular line	
V_5	Anterior axillary line (halfway between V_4 and V_6)	
V_6	Midaxillary line level with V_4	

Precordial leads, designated V_1 to V_6, provide a horizontal view of the heart's electrical activity. The horizontal plane is a horizontal or transverse cut through the middle of the heart from side to side, dividing it into upper and lower portions. The electrical activity is viewed superiorly or inferiorly.

Horizontal plane

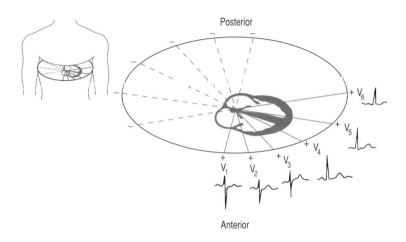

Leads V_1 to V_4 provide information about electrical activity generated anteriorly; leads V_5 and V_6 provide data on electrical activity generated laterally. Lead V_1 is commonly used in advanced ECG monitoring to distinguish bundle branch blocks and ectopy from aberrant rhythms. However, continuously monitoring a client with a V_1 lead on a 12-lead ECG machine is not always practical when a single-lead monitoring system is available.

The 12 leads and the areas of the heart they monitor consist of the following:

Lead	View
I, aV_L, V_5, V_6	Lateral
II, III, aV_F	Inferior
V_1-V_4	Anterior
aV_R	Views only the heart's base (primarily the atria and the great vessels); does not view any heart wall

VECTORS AND CURRENT FLOW

Vectors describe the size and direction of current flow from the sinoatrial (SA) node throughout the myocardium.

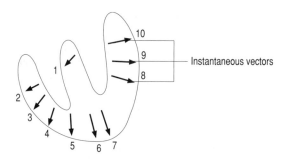

Instantaneous vectors are used to illustrate the simultaneous occurrence of all electrical forces. The sum of the instantaneous vectors can be averaged to identify a mean QRS vector.

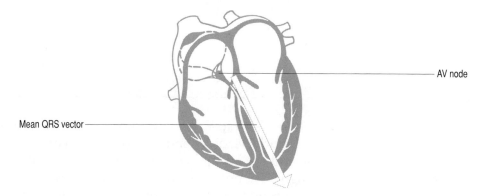

The mean QRS vector is downward and to the left because the impulse starts high in the right atrium and the main uptake of electrical forces occurs in the left ventricle. The mean QRS vector, also called the electrical axis, is the orientation of the current flow in the chest.

If the main current flow is traveling toward the positive recording electrode of a lead, the ECG records a positive QRS complex.

Current flow and the QRS complex

When current flows toward the positive recording electrode (+), the ECG shows a positive QRS complex. When current flows away from the positive recording electrode, the ECG shows a negative QRS complex. An equiphasic QRS complex occurs when the current flows perpendicularly to the recording electrode.

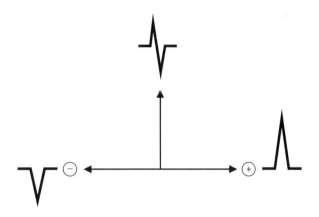

The varying appearance of the QRS complex, as seen in the precordial leads of a normal ECG, is shown in *QRS complexes,* page 22.

If the main current flow is traveling away from the positive recording electrode and toward the negative electrode, the ECG records a negative QRS complex. If the current flow is perpendicular to the recording electrode, the ECG records an equiphasic (equally positive and negative) QRS complex. This explains why QRS complexes can have different shapes and sizes.

Because the mean QRS vector is down and to the left and the left ventricle takes up most of the electrical forces, the QRS complexes should become more positive moving across the precordium. The positive recording electrode in lead V_1 is located at the right sternal border. In this lead, the QRS complex should be mostly negative because the current is flowing left. Conversely, in lead V_6 the QRS complex should be mostly positive because the current is flowing right. This pattern is called good R wave progression. An interruption of current flow in the anterior wall, which occurs in a myocardial infarction, causes poor R wave progression.

QRS complexes

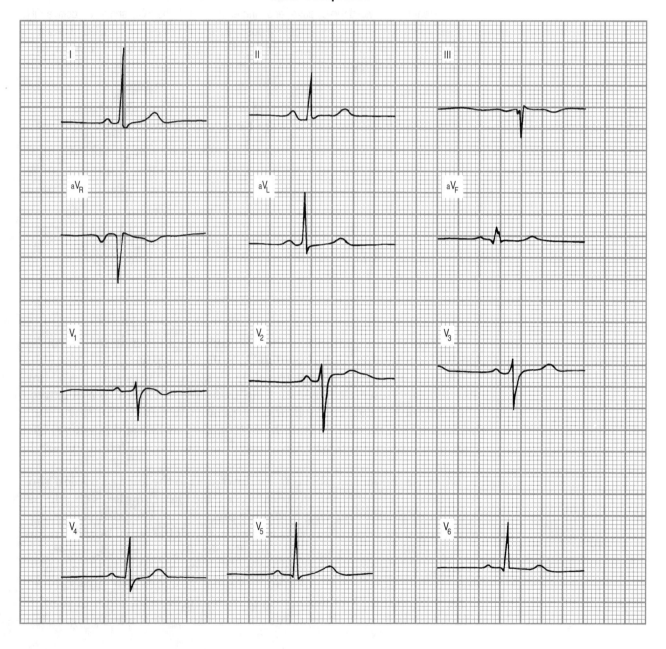

OBTAINING AN ECG

Because serial ECGs are compared to document changes in a client's condition, the recording techniques must be uniform. To ensure uniformity, the ECG is standardized, or calibrated, so that the QRS complexes are sized consistently from one recording to the next. When a standardization button is pressed, the recorder introduces 1 mV into the ECG machine; this 1 mV must measure 10 mm, or two large boxes, in height.

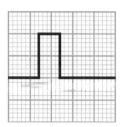

When the ECG is correctly calibrated, changes in the size of the QRS complexes are not due to inconsistencies in the recording.

To obtain accurate serial ECGs, the electrodes must be placed at the same sites. Arm leads should be placed over the wrists; leg leads, over the

---

Cardiac monitoring

Cardiac monitoring continuously records a client's heart rhythm. When a client is connected to a cardiac monitor, the nurse should follow these guidelines:

• Know the components of the monitoring system.
—The *monitor* displays the heart rate and rhythm.
—The *alarm* sounds when the heart rate falls outside the preset high and low rates or when abnormal beats occur.
—*Electrodes,* adhesive-backed disks with conductive jelly in the center, are placed on the chest to record electrical activity.
• Know which type of leads you are using. Modified chest leads include Lead I, Lead II, Lead III, Lead MCL_1, and Lead MCL_4 (MCL_1 mimics V_1).
• Prepare the client's skin properly.
—Wipe the skin with alcohol, and allow it to dry before positioning the electrodes.

—If the client has a hairy chest, shave a small patch of skin before applying the electrodes.
—Avoid placing electrodes over bony prominences.
—Watch for excoriation beneath the electrodes, and rotate the position of the electrodes as necessary.
• Watch for artifacts. Sometimes confused with an arrhythmia, these distortions of the ECG tracing may be caused by interference, such as from respirations, loose electrode or wire connections, damaged wires, electrical interference, muscle tremors, or client movement. Assess the client and check all connections before interpreting and treating as an arrhythmia.

ankles. Precordial leads should be placed as accurately as possible be-cause changes in their position will alter the data obtained from different recordings.

The electrodes must be attached securely to the skin to obtain a record-ing that is free from artifact (distortion). Electrode jelly is used to improve contact between the electrode and the skin. Skin preparation is similar to that for cardiac monitoring (see *Cardiac monitoring*, page 23). Because the limb leads of a 12-lead ECG record electrical activity in the frontal plane from a precise perspective, the client must remain supine during the pro-cedure. An upright position will alter the data produced.

COMPONENTS OF THE ECG

This discussion focuses on a normal ECG complex. Be aware that slight in-dividual variations can occur because of placement of monitoring leads on the chest and the position of the heart in the thorax. (See *Common ab-normalities of the ECG complex*, page 30.)

ECG complex The ECG complex is a visual representation of the electrical activity that occurs during one cardiac cycle. The heart's electrical activity produces waves arbitrarily labeled P, QRS, and T. Between cardiac cycles, the ECG recorder returns to a baseline called the isoelectric line. A positive wave occurs above the isoelectric line; a negative wave occurs below it. An equiphasic wave occurs equally above and below the isoelectric line.

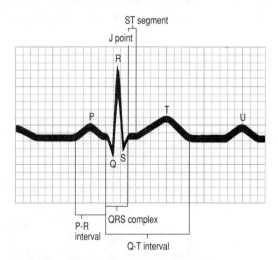

ECG paper ECG paper is graph paper that runs through the recorder at a speed of 25 mm/second, allowing the different components of the ECG complex to be measured.

The speed can be increased to 50 mm/second to examine the shapes of the ECG complexes in greater detail.

ECG paper is divided into small boxes and larger, heavy-lined boxes. Horizontal tracings across the length of the paper measure time or duration, such as the heart rate in beats/minute or the duration of the P-R interval. Vertical tracings across the width of the paper measure size or amplitude of the voltage of the ECG complex components. Horizontally, each small box measures 0.04 second. Vertically, each small box represents 1 mm in size or 0.1 mV in voltage. Each large box, which holds five smaller boxes, measures 0.20 second horizontally and 5 mm or 0.5 mV vertically. ECG paper is marked at 3-second intervals (every 15 large boxes), which aids in measuring heart rate and pauses between beats.

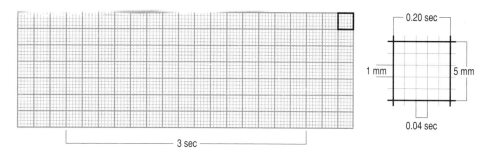

Frequently measured components of the ECG complex are the P-R interval, QRS duration, and Q-T interval. ECG calipers are recommended for measuring intervals and heart rate.

P wave The P wave depicts atrial depolarization, or the spread of the impulse from the SA node throughout the atria.

Normal P waves are positive (upright) in lead II and rounded in shape. They precede each QRS complex, indicating that the impulse is being conducted to the ventricles. Their amplitude should be less than 2.5 mm high, and their duration less than 0.11 second.

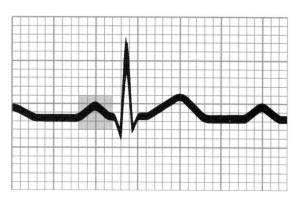

If the P waves do not look alike and are not positive in lead II, the impulse may have been initiated at a site outside the SA node. If each QRS complex is not preceded by a P wave, other sites of impulse formation or a conduction disturbance may be the cause. A P wave that is long in duration, excessively large, and not smoothly rounded may result from atrial enlargement or hypertrophy. These conditions can occur in clients with chronic obstructive pulmonary disease, pulmonary embolism, valvular disease, or congestive heart failure.

P-R interval The P-R interval corresponds to the spread of the impulse through the interatrial and internodal fibers, the atrioventricular (AV) node, the bundle of His, and the Purkinje fibers.

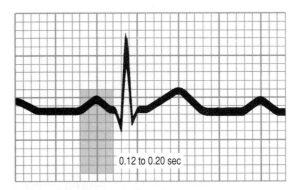

0.12 to 0.20 sec

A normal P-R interval, which is measured from the beginning of the P wave to the beginning of the QRS complex, is 0.12 to 0.20 second. A shorter interval may indicate that the impulse was initiated outside the SA node or that an accessory, faster-than-normal conduction pathway is present. A longer interval may indicate a delay in the conduction system.

QRS complex The QRS complex follows the P wave and depicts ventricular depolarization, or phase 0 of the action potential.

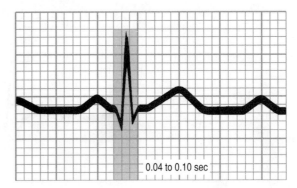

0.04 to 0.10 sec

The Q wave is the first negative wave seen after the P wave. The R wave is the first positive deflection after the Q wave, and the S wave is the first negative deflection after the R wave. Although called the QRS complex, all three waves are not always seen, because of normal or pathologic variations.

Configurations of QRS complexes

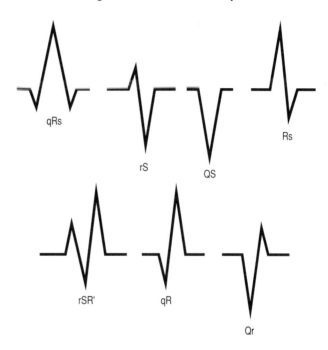

Atrial repolarization also occurs during ventricular depolarization but is obscured by the QRS complex.

A normal QRS complex, which is measured from the beginning of the Q wave to the end of the S wave, has a duration of 0.04 to 0.10 second. The J point (junction point) marks where the S wave ends and the ST segment begins.

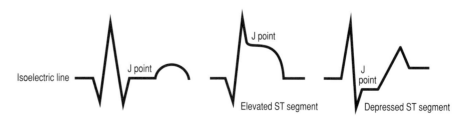

When the S wave does not end on the isoelectric line, it must be approximated down to the line. A longer-than-normal QRS complex duration indicates a ventricular conduction delay or an impulse that originated in the ventricles.

ST segment The ST segment depicts the plateau phase of the action potential, during which the myocardium is still in the absolute refractory period. The plateau phase marks the beginning of repolarization.

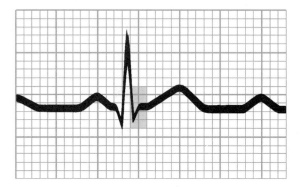

A normal ST segment initially begins at the isoelectric line, extending from the end of the S wave and gradually sloping upward to the beginning of the T wave. If the initial portion of the ST segment is depressed or flat, mild ischemia or drug effects (such as from digoxin) may be the cause. Suspect more severe myocardial ischemia if the ST segment is elevated. A 12-lead ECG should be obtained for verification.

T wave The T wave depicts the relative refractory period, or phase 3 of the action potential, and indicates ventricular repolarization.

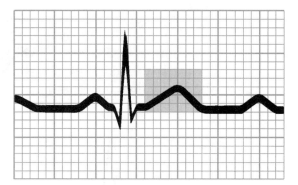

A normal T wave is smooth, rounded, and upright in most leads. An inverted T wave can be caused by myocardial injury or ventricular enlargement. If the T wave is the opposite of a prolonged QRS complex — for example, if the T wave is inverted and the QRS complex is mainly positive — ventricular ectopy or a ventricular conduction delay may be present. Peaked, tented T waves are commonly seen in clients with hyperkalemia.

The relative refractory phase depicted by the T wave is referred to as the vulnerable period because a strong stimulus at this time can precipitate an action potential.

A premature ectopic impulse that occurs during this period may initiate a reentrant arrhythmia (one in which the impulse returns to reactivate previously stimulated tissue). Such an occurrence is called an R on T phenomenon.

Q-T interval The Q-T interval — the time from ventricular depolarization to ventricular repolarization — is measured from the beginning of the Q wave to the end of the T wave on the isoelectric line.

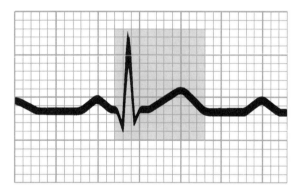

Although not routinely measured, the Q-T interval may be prolonged in clients with hypocalcemia and in those receiving antiarrhythmic medications, such as quinidine sulfate, procainamide, and disopyramide. A prolonged Q-T interval lengthens the relative refractory, or vulnerable, period, which may precipitate tachyarrhythmias (fast heart beats) if a premature stimulus occurs. The Q-T interval commonly is measured when a client begins treatment with certain antiarrhythmic drugs. The Q-T interval may be shortened in clients with hypercalcemia and in those receiving such medications as isoproterenol, a sympathomimetic drug that enhances conduction.

Common abnormalities of the ECG complex

Wave or interval	Abnormality	Etiology
P wave	Dissimilar in appearance to other P waves	• Ectopic impulse • Disturbance in atrial conduction
	Long in duration, enlarged, or not smooth and round	• Atrial hypertrophy from congestive heart failure; pulmonary or valvular disease
P-R interval	Shortened	• Ectopic impulse • Accessory conduction pathway
	Lengthened	• Atrioventricular conduction delay
QRS duration	Lengthened	• Ventricular conduction delay • Ventricular ectopy
ST segment	Flat or depressed	• Mild ischemia • Digoxin effects
	Elevated	• Myocardial ischemia
T wave	Inverted	• Myocardial injury • Ventricular enlargement
	Peaked	• Hyperkalemia
Q-T interval	Shortened	• Hypercalcemia • Effect of drugs (such as isoproterenol) that speed conduction
	Lengthened	• Hypocalcemia • Effect of drugs (such as quinidine, procainamide, and disopyramide) that slow conduction
U wave	Prominent	• Hypokalemia • Digoxin effects
	Inverted	• Ischemia

The Q-T interval varies with the heart rate: it is longer with slower heart rates and shorter with faster ones. Therefore, the Q-T interval can be measured more accurately if it is corrected for heart rate. To calculate the corrected Q-T interval, or Q-Tc, follow these steps:
• Determine the Q-T interval (as noted earlier, measure from the beginning of the Q wave to the end of the T wave).
• Determine the R-R interval (measure from the top of one R wave to the top of the next R wave).
• Divide the Q-T interval by the square root of the R-R interval. The Q-Tc should be about 0.39 second for men and 0.44 second for women. (See *Calculating the Q-Tc interval.*)

Calculating the Q–Tc interval

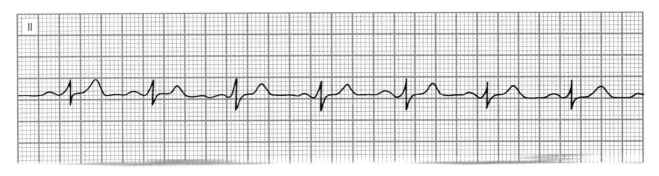

$$Q\text{-}Tc = \frac{QT\ \text{interval}}{\sqrt{R\text{-}R\ \text{interval}}}$$

$$Q\text{-}Tc = \frac{0.40\ \text{sec}}{\sqrt{0.80\ \text{sec}}}$$

$$Q\text{-}Tc = \frac{0.40}{0.894}$$

$$Q\text{-}Tc = 0.447\ \text{sec}$$

U wave   The U wave, which is not always present, signifies Purkinje fiber repolarization.

A normal U wave, smaller than the T wave it follows, usually is more apparent with a slow heart rate. A prominent U wave may indicate either hypokalemia or the electrophysiologic effect of digoxin on the conduction system. Suspect ischemia if both the U wave and the T wave are inverted.

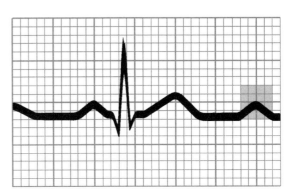

MEASURING HEART RATE

Heart rate can be measured in several ways, depending on whether the client's rhythm is regular or irregular. (For information on rhythm measurement, see *How to determine rhythm*.) The techniques discussed in this section can be used to determine ventricular and atrial rates. When calculating ventricular rates, measure R-R intervals; when calculating atrial rates, measure P-P intervals.

How to determine rhythm

You can use one of two methods to determine atrial or ventricular rhythm.

Paper and pencil method

Place the ECG strip on a flat surface; then position the straight edge of a piece of paper along the strip's baseline. Now move the paper up slightly so the straight edge is near the peak of the P waves. With a pencil, make dots on the paper at the first two P waves; this is the P-P interval. Now move the paper across the strip from left to right, lining up the two dots with succeeding P-P intervals. If the distance for each P-P interval is the same, the atrial rhythm is regular. If the distance varies, the rhythm is irregular.

Using the same method, measure the distance between the R waves of consecutive QRS complexes (the R-R interval) to determine whether the ventricular rhythm is regular or irregular.

Calipers method

With the ECG strip on a flat surface, place one point of the ECG calipers on the peak of the first P wave. Then adjust the caliper legs so the other point is on the peak of the next P wave. This distance is the P-P interval. Now move the calipers, placing the first point on the peak of the second P wave. Note whether the other point is on the peak of the third P wave.

Check succeeding P-P intervals in this manner. If all the intervals are the same, the atrial rhythm is regular; if the intervals vary, the rhythm is irregular.

Using the same method, measure the R-R intervals of consecutive QRS complexes to determine whether the ventricular rhythm is regular or irregular.

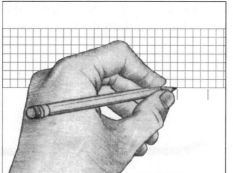
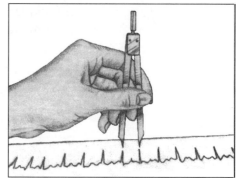

Irregular rhythms   To measure the heart rate of a client with irregular rhythms, count the number of QRS complexes in a 6-second strip (two marked-off 3-second intervals) and multiply by 10. This calculation provides an approximate heart rate in beats per minute. (*Note:* All practice examples and self-tests in this book use 6-second strips.)

Regular rhythms   To measure the heart rate of a client with regular rhythms, use the sequence, or triplicate, method. On a strip of ECG paper, draw a dark line at the top of one large box (indicated by a capital A in the next strip). On each of the following large boxes, mark 300, 150, 100, 75, 60, 50, 43, 38, 33, and 30.

   Using calipers, measure several R-R intervals to ensure that the rhythm is regular. Then bring the calipers back to the dark line, placing one end of the caliper on the line and noting where the other end falls among the number sequence. For example, if the end of the caliper lands on the box marked 150, the heart rate is 150 beats/minute.

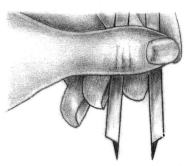

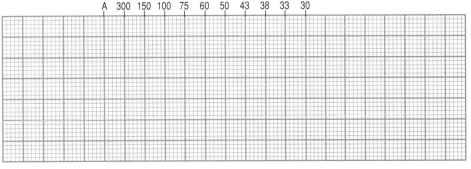

   What if the caliper falls between two boxes — for example, two small boxes after the box marked 75 but not on the 60 box? Subtract 60 from 75, leaving 15. Then divide 15 by 5 (the number of small boxes in a large box), leaving 3. Therefore, each small box between the 60 and 75 interval represents an increment of 3 beats/minute. So two small boxes (2 x 3 = 6) after 75 indicates a heart rate of 69 beats/minute (75 – 6 = 69).

These increments are different for each set of intervals. For example, each small box between 100 and 150 is an increment of 10 beats/minute (150 – 100 = 50; 50 divided by 5 = 10). Although this method is difficult to master at first, it becomes easier with practice. (Take the self-test in Chapter 3 to practice measuring intervals and heart rate.)

A less difficult method of calculating heart rate is to count the number of small boxes in one R-R interval and divide that number into 1,500 (the number of small boxes in a 1-minute rhythm strip). Another method is to count the number of large boxes in one R-R interval and divide that number into 300 (the number of large boxes in a 1-minute rhythm strip). This division has already been done in the following rate conversion tables.

Rate conversion table using small boxes

Small boxes in R-R interval	Heart rate	Small boxes in R-R interval	Heart rate	Small boxes in R-R interval	Heart rate
4	375	20	75	36	42
5	300	21	71	37	40
6	250	22	68	38	39
7	214	23	65	39	38
8	188	24	62	40	38
9	167	25	60	41	37
10	150	26	58	42	36
11	136	27	55	43	35
12	125	28	54	44	34
13	115	29	52	45	33
14	107	30	50	46	33
15	100	31	48	47	32
16	94	32	47	48	31
17	88	33	45	49	31
18	83	34	44	50	30
19	79	35	43		

Rate conversion table using large boxes

Large boxes in R-R interval	Heart rate	Large boxes in R-R interval	Heart rate	Large boxes in R-R interval	Heart rate
1	300	5	60	9	33
2	150	6	50	10	30
3	100	7	43		
4	75	8	38		

SYSTEMATIC APPROACH TO ARRHYTHMIA INTERPRETATION

To avoid overlooking an important aspect of arrhythmia interpretation, use the following format when interpreting a rhythm strip:

ECG characteristics

P wave *Configuration:* Do all the P waves look alike? Are they upright in lead II? Is one P wave seen for each QRS complex? Does the P wave precede the QRS complex?
Rate: What is the atrial rate?
Rhythm: Is the P-P interval regular?

P-R interval What is the P-R interval? Does it remain the same throughout the strip?

QRS complex *Configuration:* Do all the QRS complexes look alike? Does a QRS complex follow each P wave?
Rate: What is the ventricular rate?
Rhythm: Is the R-R interval regular?
Duration: What is the QRS interval?

Interpretation Is an arrhythmia present? Which kind?

Treatment What medical treatment should be anticipated? Which medications are usually needed for this arrhythmia? Is cardioversion or defibrillation warranted? Should CPR be initiated?

Nursing implications What nursing actions are required? Should the client's activity level be restricted? Is the client positioned properly (for instance, a supine position to combat hypotension or a high-Fowler's position to counter dyspnea)?

Finally, consider the arrhythmia's severity, the client's condition, and the monitoring equipment being used. For instance, is the arrhythmia significant? Does the client's physical appearance provide clues to a serious problem? Is the ECG monitor properly connected? Is the client doing anything (such as brushing teeth) that might interfere with proper monitoring? Developing the habit of asking such questions enables you to follow a systematic approach to arrhythmia interpretation until it becomes second nature.

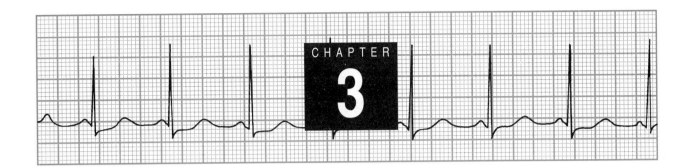

Sinus Arrhythmias

Although sinus rhythms originate normally in the sinoatrial (SA) node, some are arrhythmic in rate (such as sinus bradycardia and sinus tachycardia) and others in rhythm (such as sinus arrhythmia). These abnormal rhythms can be benign or have serious consequences, such as those of extremely slow sinus bradycardia.

This chapter focuses on interpretation of the major sinus arrhythmias, including sinus bradycardia, sinus tachycardia, sinus arrhythmia, and sinus arrest and exit block. For each rhythm, the text describes ECG characteristics, effects on the client, standard treatments, and implications for the nurse. To enhance learning, practice examples appear after the discussion of each arrhythmia, and the chapter concludes with three self-tests.

NORMAL SINUS RHYTHM

Normal sinus rhythm reflects the heart's normal electrical activity. The impulse originates in the SA node (the heart's pacemaker, located in the right atrium) and travels to the atrioventricular (AV) node, the right and left bundle branches, and finally to the Purkinje fibers (see *Conduction and innervation*).

Conduction and innervation

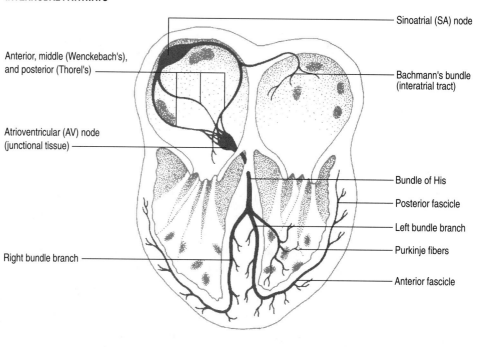

INTERNODAL PATHWAYS

Anterior, middle (Wenckebach's), and posterior (Thorel's)

Atrioventricular (AV) node (junctional tissue)

Right bundle branch

Sinoatrial (SA) node

Bachmann's bundle (interatrial tract)

Bundle of His

Posterior fascicle

Left bundle branch

Purkinje fibers

Anterior fascicle

In normal sinus rhythm, the atria contract first, then the ventricles; this sequence produces efficient heartbeats.

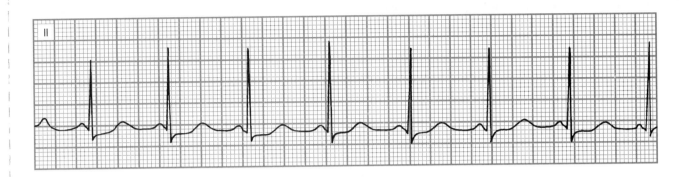

ECG characteristics

P wave *Configuration.* The P waves should be upright in lead II, with one P wave preceding each QRS complex. All P waves should be identical.
Rate: The atrial rate should be between 60 and 100 beats/minute.
Rhythm: The P-P interval should be regular, although differences of up to 0.12 second are considered normal.

P-R interval The P-R interval remains between 0.12 and 0.20 second.

QRS complex *Configuration:* Each QRS complex should be preceded by a P wave. All QRS complexes should be identical throughout the strip.
Rate: The ventricular rate should be between 60 and 100 beats/minute.
Rhythm: The R-R interval should be regular, although differences of up to 0.12 second are considered normal.
Duration: The duration of the QRS complex can be normal or wide (prolonged). A normal QRS complex indicates normal conduction throughout the bundle branches. A wide QRS complex indicates abnormal conduction, perhaps caused by a bundle branch block. (Note: A bundle branch block cannot be diagnosed with one-lead monitors; consequently, the text refers to a wide QRS complex as an intraventricular conduction defect or bundle branch block pattern.)

Effects on the client Because normal sinus rhythm is the desired rhythm, no adverse events should occur. However, some clients with cardiovascular disease may not have the cardiac reserve to tolerate rates at either extreme of the normal range (60 to 100 beats/minute). In these clients, cardiac output may decrease if the heart rate drops too low, or cardiac filling may decrease if the heart rate becomes too high.

Treatment No treatment is needed for this rhythm. However, any client with a cardiac monitor, even a client with a normal sinus rhythm, should be watched closely.

Nursing implications
- Determine whether this rhythm is an effective one for the client. A client with cardiovascular disease who cannot tolerate high or low heart rates may experience hypotension, dizziness, or chest pain.
- If a client converts to a normal sinus rhythm from an arrhythmia, as in cardiac arrest, ensure that the client has an effective pulse rate and blood pressure.

Practice example   Carefully study the ECG strip in the following example; then test your rhythm interpretation skills by filling in the blank lines with the appropriate information, using the knowledge you have obtained from this and earlier chapters. Check your responses against the correct answers provided later in this chapter on page 54.

PRACTICE EXAMPLE

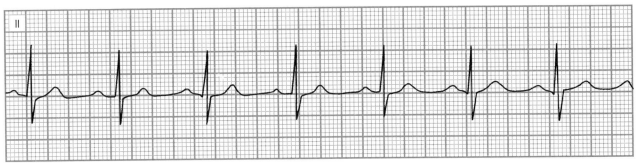

ECG characteristics

P wave   *Configuration:* _____

_____

Rate: _____

_____

Rhythm: _____

_____

P-R interval _____

_____

QRS complex   *Configuration:* _____

_____

Rate: _____

_____

Rhythm: _____

_____

Duration: _____

_____

Interpretation _____

_____

SINUS BRADYCARDIA

In sinus bradycardia, the impulse originates in the SA node at a rate slower than that of a normal sinus rhythm. The impulse then travels down the conduction system normally. Although sinus bradycardia has many causes, it also can be a normal variant. For instance, an athlete may have a slow heart rate because a well-conditioned heart has an unusually efficient stroke volume (the amount of blood ejected with each beat). Sinus bradycardia also can result from a decreased metabolic rate caused by hypothyroidism, hypothermia, or sleep.

Because an increase in parasympathetic tone stimulates the vagus nerve to slow the heart, sinus bradycardia can occur with vomiting, increased intracranial pressure, vasovagal maneuvers, and carotid sinus massage. Conversely, a decrease or interruption of sympathetic tone, as seen in spinal cord injury, also can slow the heart rate. This rhythm may occur during an acute inferior wall myocardial infarction or from the administration of cardiac medications, such as digoxin, verapamil, and propranolol. Sinus bradycardia also can be a symptom of sinus node disease.

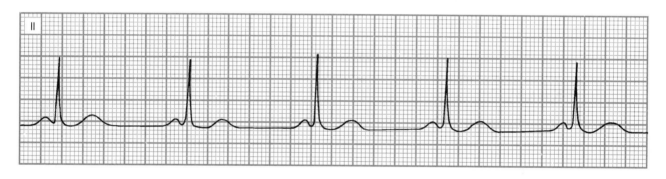

ECG characteristics

P wave   *Configuration:* The P waves should be upright in lead II, with one P wave preceding each QRS complex. All P waves should be identical.
Rate: The atrial rate is less than 60 beats/minute.
Rhythm: The P-P interval should be regular.

P-R interval   The P-R interval remains between 0.12 and 0.20 second.

QRS complex   *Configuration:* Each QRS complex should be preceded by a P wave. All QRS complexes should be identical throughout the strip.
Rate: The ventricular rate is less than 60 beats/minute.
Rhythm: The R-R interval should be regular.
Duration: The QRS complex can be normal or wide.

Effects on the client   How the rhythm affects the client depends on the slowness of the rate. Some people, especially athletes, can tolerate low heart rates without symptoms. However, if the rate becomes slow enough to decrease cardiac output significantly, hypotension and syncope may occur.

Treatment   If sinus bradycardia produces symptoms, the treatment of choice is the parasympatholytic drug atropine sulfate, which prevents the vagus nerve from slowing the heart. The standard dosage is 0.5 mg by I.V. push every 5 minutes until the bradycardia resolves or a maximum dose of 2 mg has been administered. If the arrhythmia still does not resolve, a transvenous or transcutaneous pacemaker may be needed. Until the pacemaker is inserted, a continuous infusion of isoproterenol (Isuprel), a sympathomimetic drug, should be given at a rate of 2 to 10 mcg/minute.

Nursing implications
- Because many cases of sinus bradycardia are asymptomatic, carefully assess the client before initiating therapy; the treatment itself can cause complications.
- Clients at risk for sinus bradycardia include those receiving multiple cardiac medications that depress the SA node.
- Because sinus bradycardia can result from carotid sinus massage (a treatment for suppressing or diagnosing certain tachyarrhythmias), this procedure should be performed only by a physician skilled in the technique and only in a monitored situation in which emergency medications are readily available.
- When initiating treatment for symptomatic sinus bradycardia, be sure to administer the correct dose. Atropine sulfate at doses of 0.25 mg exerts a sympatholytic effect and can further decrease the heart rate. Isoproterenol is a potentially dangerous drug because it can precipitate lethal ventricular arrhythmias.
- Administer medications only if necessary, and always use a volumetric infusion pump for accurate drug delivery. If ventricular arrhythmias occur, immediately discontinue the isoproterenol infusion.

Practice example   Carefully study the ECG strip in the following example; then test your rhythm interpretation skills by filling in the blank lines with the appropriate information, using the knowledge you have obtained from this and earlier chapters. Check your responses against the correct answers provided later in this chapter on page 54.

PRACTICE EXAMPLE

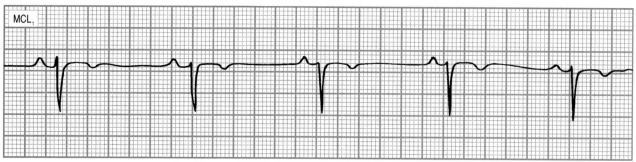

ECG characteristics

P wave *Configuration:*

_____

_____

Rate:

_____

_____

Rhythm:

_____

_____

P-R interval

_____

_____

QRS complex *Configuration:*

_____

_____

Rate:

_____

_____

Rhythm:

_____

_____

Duration:

_____

_____

Interpretation

_____

_____

SINUS TACHYCARDIA

In sinus tachycardia, the impulse originates in the SA node at a rate faster than that of a normal sinus rhythm. The impulse then travels down the conduction system normally. This arrhythmia can be caused by stimulation of the sympathetic nervous system from fear, pain, or the effect of sympathomimetic drugs; an elevated metabolic rate caused by hyperthyroidism, fever, or exercise; or a decrease in the oxygen-carrying capacity of the blood, as seen in clients with anemia, hypoxia, and respiratory disease. Sinus tachycardia is normal in children (see *Normal heart rates in children*).

Normal heart rates In children

Age	Heart rate (beats/minute)	Average rate (beats/minute)
Newborn to 3 months	85 to 205	140
3 months to 2 years	100 to 190	130
2 to 10 years	60 to 140	80
Older than 10 years	50 to 100	75

Source: Chameides, L., ed. *Textbook of Pediatric Advanced Life Support.* American Heart Association, 1988.

Tachycardia is a compensatory mechanism in states of decreased cardiac output, such as shock or congestive heart failure. In these cases, the heart rate increases to maintain cardiac output in the face of falling stroke volume.

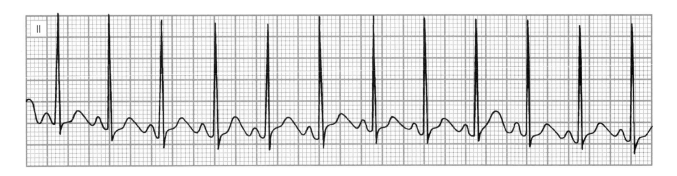

ECG characteristics

P wave *Configuration:* The P waves should be upright in lead II, with one P wave preceding each QRS complex. All P waves should be identical. At faster heart rates, the P wave may not be visible if it is buried in the preceding T wave.

Rate: The atrial rate should be between 100 and 160 beats/minute.
Rhythm: The P-P interval should be regular, although differences of up to 0.12 second are considered normal.

P-R interval   The P-R interval remains between 0.12 and 0.20 second.

QRS complex   *Configuration:* Each QRS complex should be preceded by a P wave. All QRS complexes should be identical throughout the strip.
Rate: The ventricular rate should be between 100 and 160 beats/minute.
Rhythm: The R-R interval should be regular, although differences of up to 0.12 second are considered normal.
Duration: The QRS complex can be normal or wide.

Effects on the client   The client may complain of chest palpitations or fluttering. Because the coronary arteries fill during diastole, which is shortened in tachycardia, chest pain may result from a persistently rapid rate. A susceptible client with a history of cardiac disease also may experience chest pain. At faster rates, cardiac output may diminish, causing hypotension and decreased cerebral perfusion.

Treatment   Sinus tachycardia resolves once the underlying cause is treated. For example, if a client experiences sinus tachycardia because of pain, administration of pain medication should end the arrhythmia. Relaxation techniques also are effective; these independent nursing interventions are useful adjuncts to treatment if the sinus tachycardia results from pain or fear. The physician may perform carotid sinus massage to differentiate sinus tachycardia from other tachyarrhythmias. Carotid sinus massage temporarily slows the heart rate.

Nursing implications   • Assess the client for chest pain, rales, an S_3 heart sound, and jugular vein distention.
• If a client experiences an acute myocardial infarction, sinus tachycardia may enlarge the infarcted area because the faster heart rate increases oxygen demand. Congestive heart failure also can result if cardiac output decreases.

Practice example   Carefully study the ECG strip in the following example; then test your rhythm interpretation skills by filling in the blank lines with the appropriate information, using the knowledge you have obtained from this and earlier chapters. Check your responses against the correct answers provided later in this chapter on pages 54 and 55.

PRACTICE EXAMPLE

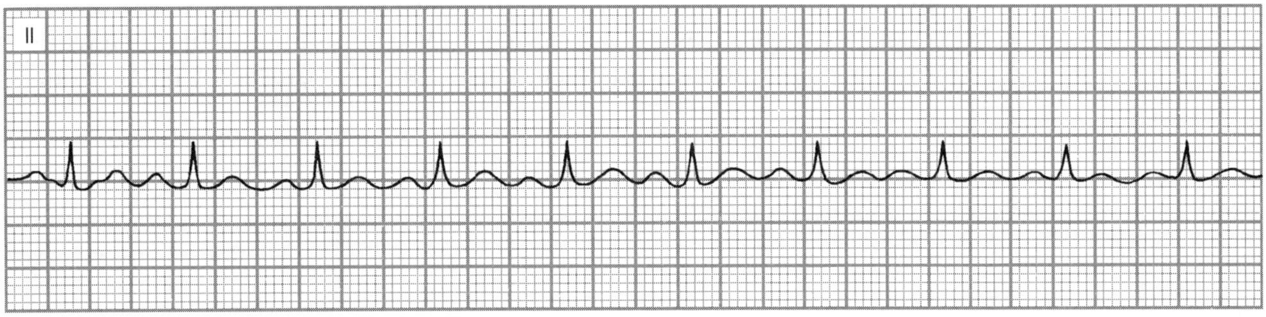

ECG characteristics

P wave   *Configuration:*

_____

Rate:

_____

Rhythm:

_____

P-R interval

_____

QRS complex   *Configuration:*

_____

Rate:

_____

Rhythm:

_____

Duration:

_____

Interpretation

_____

SINUS ARRHYTHMIA

In sinus arrhythmia, the impulse originates in the SA node at an irregular rate, then travels down the conduction system normally. This benign arrhythmia is commonly related to vagal inhibition caused by respiration.

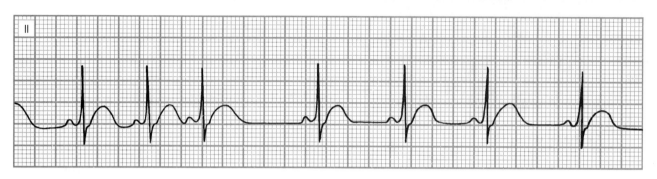

ECG characteristics

P wave *Configuration:* The P waves should be upright in lead II, with one P wave preceding each QRS complex. All P waves should be identical.
Rate: The atrial rate may vary from 60 to 100 beats/minute.
Rhythm: The P-P interval is irregular.

P-R interval The P-R interval remains between 0.12 and 0.20 second.

QRS complex *Configuration:* Each QRS complex should be preceded by a P wave. All QRS complexes should be identical throughout the strip.
Rate: The ventricular rate may vary from 60 to 100 beats/minute.
Rhythm: The R-R interval is irregular, increasing with inspiration and decreasing with expiration. The difference between the shortest and longest R-R interval is greater than 0.12 second. To calculate this difference, measure the shortest R-R interval with calipers. Then place the calipers — without changing the distance measured — at the first QRS complex of the longest R-R interval. Count the distance in small boxes from the second point of the caliper to the second QRS complex in the longest R-R interval. This number is the difference between the shortest and longest R-R intervals.
Duration: The QRS complex can be normal or wide.

Effects on the client This arrhythmia is usually asymptomatic. If the arrhythmia is severe, palpitations and dizziness may occur.

Treatment No treatment is needed.

Nursing implications Be careful not to confuse a markedly irregular sinus arrhythmia with a more severe arrhythmia, such as atrial fibrillation or an AV block.

Practice example   Carefully study the ECG strip in the following example; then test your rhythm interpretation skills by filling in the blank lines with the appropriate information, using the knowledge you have obtained from this and earlier chapters. Check your responses against the correct answers provided later in this chapter on page 55.

PRACTICE EXAMPLE

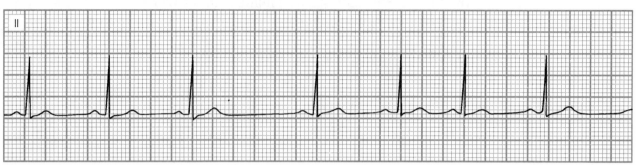

ECG characteristics

P wave *Configuration:* _____

_____

Rate: _____

_____

Rhythm: _____

_____

P-R interval _____

_____

QRS complex *Configuration:* _____

_____

Rate: _____

_____

Rhythm: _____

_____

Duration: _____

_____

Interpretation _____

_____

SINUS ARREST AND EXIT BLOCK

Sinus arrest and exit block — two separate arrhythmias with different pathophysiologies — are discussed together here because distinguishing between them is sometimes difficult and because their treatment and clinical significance are the same.

In sinus arrest, the SA node fails to initiate an impulse as a result of depressed activity. In sinus exit block, the impulse is initiated by the SA node but is not conducted to the atria because of a block in the conduction system. These arrhythmias may result from increased vagal tone or depressed automaticity and conduction caused by certain medications, such as digoxin. Cardiac diseases that impair or destroy the conduction system, including myocardial infarction or myocarditis, also can depress automaticity.

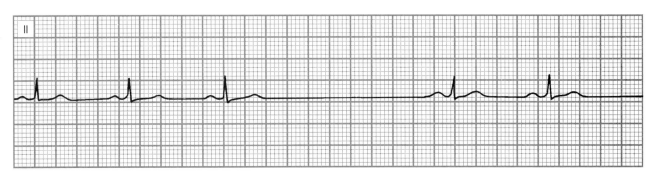

ECG characteristics

P wave   *Configuration:* The P waves should be upright in lead II, with one P wave preceding each QRS complex. All P waves should be identical. P waves are not visible when the entire ECG complex is dropped (absent).
Rate: The atrial rate may vary but usually is less than 60 beats/minute when the ECG complex is absent.
Rhythm: The P-P interval should be regular except during the pauses.

P-R interval   The P-R interval is usually normal (0.12 to 0.20 second) unless another condition, such as a first-degree AV block, exists.

QRS complex   *Configuration:* Each QRS complex should be preceded by a P wave. All QRS complexes should be identical throughout the strip. However, if the pause is long enough, escape beats from the AV node or ventricle may appear. QRS complexes are not seen when the entire ECG complex is dropped.
Rate: The ventricular rate may vary but is usually less than 60 beats/minute during the pauses.
Rhythm: The R-R interval should be regular except during the pauses. In sinus arrest, the rhythm resets after the pause, and the length of the pause

is not a multiple of the underlying R-R interval. In sinus exit block, the pause *is* a multiple of the underlying R-R interval, because the SA node continues to discharge and the rhythm does not reset.

Duration: The QRS complex can be normal or, if the pause is long enough, wide.

Effects on the client These rhythms may be undetected if the pauses are short. Long pauses can cause hypotension, dizziness, and syncope.

Treatment If the sinus arrest or exit block is symptomatic, the treatment of choice is the parasympatholytic drug atropine sulfate, which prevents the vagus nerve from slowing the heartbeat. The dosage is 0.5 mg by I.V. push every 5 minutes until the arrhythmia resolves or a maximum dose of 2 mg has been administered. If the sinus arrest or exit block still does not resolve, a temporary pacemaker is indicated. Until the pacemaker is inserted, a continuous infusion of isoproterenol (Isuprel), a sympathomimetic drug, should be given at a rate of 2 to 10 mcg/minute. If the conduction system is permanently impaired and the pauses are longer than 3 seconds, a permanent pacemaker is necessary.

Nursing implications
• Assess the client for digoxin overdose.
• Withhold all medications (such as digoxin and propranolol) that depress SA node activity or sinus conduction.

Practice example Carefully study the ECG strip in the following example; then test your rhythm interpretation skills by filling in the blank lines with the appropriate information, using the knowledge you have obtained from this and earlier chapters. Check your responses against the correct answers provided later in this chapter on pages 55 and 56.

PRACTICE EXAMPLE

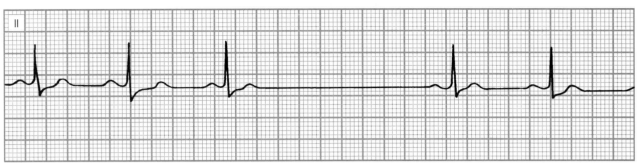

ECG characteristics

P wave   *Configuration:* _____

_____

Rate: _____

_____

Rhythm: _____

_____

P-R interval   _____

_____

QRS complex   *Configuration:* _____

_____

Rate: _____

_____

Rhythm: _____

_____

Duration: _____

_____

Interpretation   _____

_____

ANSWERS TO PRACTICE EXAMPLES

NORMAL SINUS RHYTHM

ECG characteristics

P wave — *Configuration:* All upright and identical, with one P wave preceding each QRS complex
Rate: 72 beats/minute
Rhythm: Regular

P-R interval — 0.20 second

QRS complex — *Configuration:* All normal and alike, with each QRS complex preceded by a P wave
Rate: 72 beats/minute
Rhythm: Regular
Duration: 0.10 second

Interpretation — Normal sinus rhythm

SINUS BRADYCARDIA

ECG characteristics

P wave — *Configuration:* All upright and identical, with one P wave preceding each QRS complex
Rate: 48 beats/minute
Rhythm: Regular

P-R interval — 0.20 second

QRS complex — *Configuration:* All normal and alike, with each QRS complex preceded by a P wave
Rate: 48 beats/minute
Rhythm: Regular
Duration: 0.08 second

Interpretation — Sinus bradycardia

SINUS TACHYCARDIA

ECG characteristics

P wave — *Configuration:* All upright and identical, with one P wave preceding each QRS complex
Rate: 100 beats/minute
Rhythm: Regular

P-R interval   0.20 second

QRS complex   Configuration: All normal and alike, with each QRS complex preceded by a P wave
Rate: 100 beats/minute
Rhythm: Regular
Duration: 0.08 second

Interpretation   Sinus tachycardia

SINUS ARRHYTHMIA

ECG characteristics
P wave   Configuration: All upright and identical, with one P wave preceding each QRS complex
Rate: Approximately 70 beats/minute (using the 6-second strip method)
Rhythm: The P-P interval is irregular, with 0.58 second between the shortest and longest interval

P-R interval   0.18 second

QRS complex   Configuration: All normal and alike, with each QRS complex preceded by a P wave
Rate: Approximately 70 beats/minute (using the 6-second strip method)
Rhythm: The R-R interval is irregular, with 0.58 second between the shortest and longest interval
Duration: 0.06 second

Interpretation   Sinus arrhythmia

SINUS ARREST AND EXIT BLOCK

ECG characteristics
P wave   Configuration: All upright and identical, with one P wave preceding each QRS complex
Rate: Approximately 50 beats/minute (using the 6-second strip method)
Rhythm: Regular, except for the pause caused by the dropped ECG complex between the 3rd and 4th impulses

P-R interval   0.20 second

QRS complex   *Configuration:* All normal and alike, with each QRS complex preceded by a P wave
Rate: Approximately 50 beats/minute (using the 6-second strip method)
Rhythm: Regular, except for the pause due to the dropped ECG complex between the 3rd and 4th impulses. The pause is not a multiple of the underlying R-R interval.
Duration: 0.08 second

Interpretation   Sinus arrest

SELF – TESTS

You can verify your understanding of the material presented in this chapter by completing the following self-tests. Like the practice examples, the self-tests will assess your knowledge of ECG characteristics and rhythm interpretation. Additionally, they will measure what you know about treatments and nursing implications for each arrhythmia. Complete all three self-tests in this chapter before comparing your responses to the correct answers in Appendix A, pages 201 and 202.

SELF – TEST 1

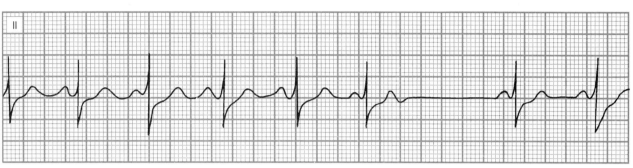

ECG characteristics

        P wave   *Configuration:*

                    Rate:

                    Rhythm:

    P-R interval

    QRS complex   *Configuration:*

                    Rate:

                    Rhythm:

                    Duration:

Interpretation _____

_____

Treatment _____

_____

_____

_____

_____

_____

Nursing implications _____

_____

_____

_____

_____

_____

SELF – TEST 2

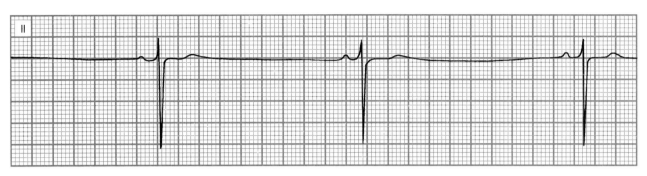

ECG characteristics

P wave   *Configuration:*

_____

Rate:

_____

Rhythm:

_____

P-R interval

_____

_____

QRS complex   *Configuration:*

_____

Rate:

_____

Rhythm:

_____

Duration:

_____

Interpretation

_____

_____

Treatment

_____

_____

_____

_____

_____

Nursing implications

_____

_____

_____

_____

_____

SELF – TEST 3

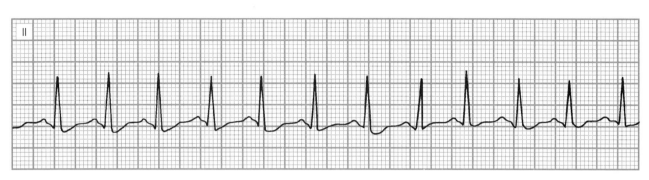

ECG characteristics

P wave   *Configuration:*
_____

_____

Rate:
_____

_____

Rhythm:
_____

_____

P-R interval
_____

_____

QRS complex   *Configuration:*
_____

_____

Rate:
_____

_____

Rhythm:
_____

_____

Duration:
_____

_____

Interpretation _____

_____

Treatment _____

_____

_____

_____

_____

_____

Nursing implications _____

_____

_____

_____

_____

_____

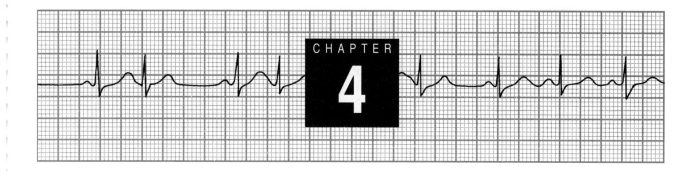

4

Atrial Arrhythmias

Most atrial arrhythmias result from enhanced automaticity, which causes an ectopic site (one outside the normal conduction system) to initiate an impulse spontaneously. Ectopic sites tend to fire quickly, producing a rapid atrial rate. Not all of these impulses are conducted to the ventricles because of the normal delay at the atrioventricular (AV) node, which allows the ventricles to fill with blood. This prevents the development of a rapid ventricular rate that could cause chest pain and hypotension.

This chapter focuses on interpretation of the major atrial arrhythmias, including premature atrial contraction, paroxysmal and nonparoxysmal atrial tachycardia, atrial flutter, atrial fibrillation, wandering atrial pacemaker, and multifocal atrial tachycardia. For each rhythm, the text describes ECG characteristics, effects on the client, standard treatments, and implications for the nurse. To enhance learning, practice examples appear after the discussion of each arrhythmia, and the chapter concludes with four self-tests.

PREMATURE ATRIAL CONTRACTION

A premature atrial contraction (PAC) is an ectopic beat caused by enhanced automaticity in the atrial tissue. It occurs in addition to the client's normal underlying rhythm. This early beat may travel down the conduction system normally and produce a QRS complex similar to the client's normal one. The early beat also may travel down the conduction system abnormally; that is, it may travel down one bundle branch and become blocked in the other, producing an abnormal QRS complex. This is called aberrant conduction. The illustration below shows the location of an abnormal atrial impulse. Arrows indicate the direction the impulse may travel.

Atrial origin of premature impulse

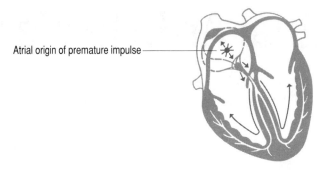

Sometimes, the PAC occurs so soon after the preceding impulse that ventricular tissue is still in the refractory phase, and the PAC is not conducted to the ventricles. This is called a blocked or nonconducted PAC. PACs usually occur from irritation of the atrial tissue, which can be caused by ingestion of caffeine or alcohol; stress; hypoxia; and rheumatic, valvular, pulmonary, or ischemic heart disease. Hypokalemia, digoxin toxicity, and theophylline therapy also can cause PACs.

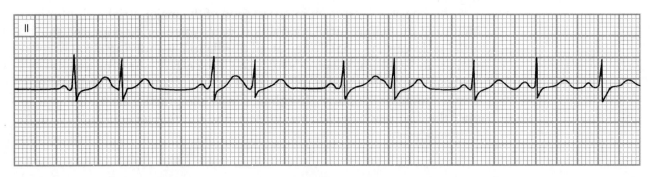

ECG characteristics

P wave   *Configuration:* The P wave of the PAC (called the P prime or P') is usually upright in lead II but looks different from the P wave of the client's under-

lying rhythm. If the PAC occurs soon after the preceding impulse, the P' may be buried in or seen as an extra hump on the preceding T wave.
Rate: The atrial rate varies, depending on the underlying rhythm.
Rhythm: The P-P interval should be irregular because of the early beat. However, the underlying P-P interval may appear regular. Because the PAC occurs prematurely, it usually resets the client's underlying rhythm so that the impulse following the PAC does not come when expected. This is called a noncompensatory pause.

P-R interval   The P-R interval varies between that of the client's underlying rhythm and the PAC. The P-R interval between PACs also may vary if multiple ectopic sites are involved.

QRS complex   *Configuration:* Each QRS complex of the PAC should follow a P wave unless the PAC is blocked or not conducted. The QRS complex of the PAC is similar to the underlying QRS complex unless the beat is aberrantly conducted.
Rate: The ventricular rate varies, depending on the underlying rhythm.
Rhythm: The R-R interval is irregular because the premature beat arrives early. However, the underlying R-R interval may be regular. Different patterns emerge in multiple PACs, such as atrial bigeminy (one normal beat followed by a PAC), atrial trigeminy (two normal beats followed by a PAC), or atrial quadrigeminy (three normal beats followed by a PAC).
Duration: The QRS complex can be normal or wide, depending on whether the client's underlying QRS duration is prolonged or the PAC is aberrantly conducted.

Effects on the client   Infrequent PACs may go undetected by the client or may elicit complaints of palpitations. Frequent PACs may be a precursor of more severe atrial arrhythmias, such as atrial fibrillation or tachycardia. In clients with limited cardiac reserve, such as those with ischemic heart disease, frequent PACs can decrease cardiac output and lead to congestive heart failure.

Treatment   Infrequent PACs usually require no treatment. If treatment is needed, the best approach is to eliminate the cause (for example, caffeine). Pharmacologic therapy may include:
- digoxin 0.25 mg I.V. or by mouth every 6 hours for four doses as a loading dose, then 0.25 mg daily. Decrease the dose if quinidine is to be added, because quinidine increases serum digoxin levels.
- quinidine sulfate 200 mg by mouth or intramuscularly every 3 to 4 hours or quinidine gluconate 324 mg every 6 to 8 hours. This antiarrhythmic agent acts on both the atria and the ventricles.
- procainamide hydrochloride 250 to 500 mg by mouth every 3 hours. The oral dose of the slow-release form (Procan SR) is 500 mg to 1 g every

6 hours. This antiarrhythmic agent acts on both the atria and the ventricles.

Nursing implications
- Assess a client with PACs for potential underlying causes, and monitor serum potassium and digoxin levels.
- Assess a client with ischemic heart disease for signs and symptoms of congestive heart failure.
- Anticipate more severe atrial arrhythmias if PACs become more frequent.
- Teach the client to avoid caffeine and to use stress reduction techniques.

Practice example   Carefully study the ECG strip in the following example; then test your rhythm interpretation skills by filling in the blank lines with the appropriate information, using the knowledge you have obtained from this and earlier chapters. Check your responses against the correct answers provided later in this chapter on page 86.

PRACTICE EXAMPLE

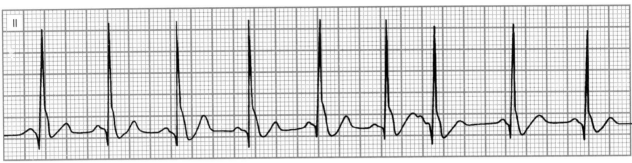

ECG characteristics

P wave   *Configuration:* _____

_____

Rate: _____

_____

Rhythm: _____

_____

P-R interval   _____

_____

QRS complex   *Configuration:* _____

_____

Rate: _____

_____

Rhythm: _____

_____

Duration: _____

_____

Interpretation   _____

_____

PAROXYSMAL AND NONPAROXYSMAL ATRIAL TACHYCARDIA

Atrial tachycardia is a tachyarrhythmia (a heart rate greater than 100 beats/minute) whose impulse formation originates in the atrial tissue. Paroxysmal atrial tachycardia, which starts and stops suddenly, is usually caused by reentry and may be initiated by a PAC; nonparoxysmal atrial tachycardia, commonly a sustained arrhythmia, is usually caused by enhanced automaticity. Sometimes, because the heart rate is so fast, P waves cannot be identified. Such cases are called supraventricular tachycardia (SVT), meaning that the impulse's origin may be in the atria or the AV node. The illustrations below show the sites of possible impulse formation. Arrows indicate the direction the impulse can travel; a circular route denotes reentry.

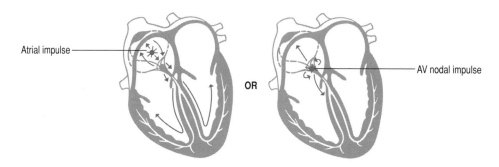

Atrial tachycardia can be caused by stress, excessive use of stimulants, an accessory conduction pathway (one that bypasses the AV node), chronic lung disease, or digoxin toxicity. When atrial tachycardia results from digoxin toxicity, some of the atrial beats are blocked at the AV node because of the drug's depressant effect. This rhythm is called atrial tachycardia with block.

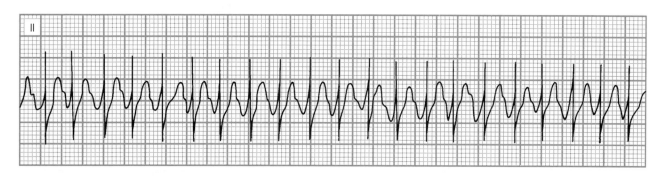

ECG characteristics

P wave   *Configuration:* P waves, if seen, are usually upright and identical. The P waves may be buried in the preceding T wave because of the fast heart

rate. At the onset of atrial tachycardia, the P waves of the tachycardia appear different from those of the underlying rhythm.
Rate: About 160 to 220 beats/minute
Rhythm: The P-P interval is usually regular.

P-R interval The P-R interval is usually normal but may not be measurable if the P waves are buried.

QRS complex *Configuration:* The QRS complexes are usually alike and may look similar to normal QRS complexes.
Rate: About 160 to 220 beats/minute
Rhythm: The R-R interval is usually regular.
Duration: QRS complex durations are usually normal but may be wide if a coincidental intraventricular conduction defect also exists or if aberrant conduction occurs.

Effects on the client Ventricular filling and cardiac output may decrease because of the fast heart rate. With a shortened diastole, coronary perfusion may be reduced, which can lead to chest pain.

Treatment Vagal stimulation, synchronized cardioversion, or overdrive pacing may control atrial tachycardia caused by reentry. Vagal stimulation can be produced through carotid sinus massage, the Valsalva maneuver, or the diving reflex (immersing a client's face in a pan of cold water). Cardioversion is the restoration of normal rhythm through electrical stimulation. Overdrive pacing involves inserting a pacemaker into the atrium to pace the myocardium at a rate higher than that of the atrial tachycardia. This procedure interrupts the circular movement of the impulse caused by the reentrant tachycardia.

Drugs can be used to control atrial tachycardia caused by reentry or enhanced automaticity. Pharmacologic therapy may include:
• digoxin 0.25 to 0.5 mg I.V.; digoxin is contraindicated in clients with an accessory conduction pathway (the drug can enhance conduction and actually speed up the arrhythmia) and in those with digoxin toxicity.
• propranolol 1 mg I.V. every 5 minutes up to a maximum dosage of 3 mg.
• verapamil 5 to 10 mg I.V.; may repeat 10 mg in 30 minutes if necessary.
• procainamide (Pronestyl) 50 mg/minute by I.V. bolus until the arrhythmia subsides, the QRS complex widens by at least 50%, or the maximum dosage of 1 g has been administered; a continuous infusion of 1 to 4 mg/minute follows.

Nursing implications • Check the client's rhythm strip for clues to what triggered the atrial tachycardia. Knowing the cause can help determine the treatment. For example, a PAC on the strip would probably indicate that the atrial

tachycardia was caused by reentry, warranting a vagal maneuver, cardioversion, or overdrive pacing.
- Make sure that resuscitative equipment is available if vagal stimulation or cardioversion is necessary; bradycardia can result from vagal stimulation, and cardioversion can be complicated by more severe arrhythmias.
- Monitor the client for chest pain and signs of congestive heart failure.
- Adminster supplemental oxygen as prescribed.
- Withhold digoxin if the client has atrial tachycardia with block or an accessory conduction pathway.

Practice example Carefully study the ECG strip in the following example; then test your rhythm interpretation skills by filling in the blank lines with the appropriate information, using the knowledge you have obtained from this and earlier chapters. Check your responses against the correct answers provided later in this chapter on page 86.

PRACTICE EXAMPLE

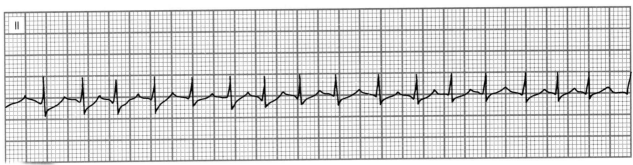

ECG characteristics

    P wave *Configuration:* _____

           _____

          Rate: _____

           _____

          Rhythm: _____

           _____

   P-R interval _____

           _____

  QRS complex *Configuration:* _____

          Rate: _____

          Rhythm: _____

          Duration: _____

           _____

  Interpretation _____

           _____

ATRIAL FLUTTER

Atrial flutter, a transient rhythm, usually precedes atrial fibrillation and is similar to the latter rhythm in impulse formation and conduction. Its rapid impulse originates in the atrial tissue, either from reentry or from enhanced automaticity. The illustration below shows the sites of possible impulse formation. Arrows indicate the direction the impulse can travel; a circular route denotes reentry.

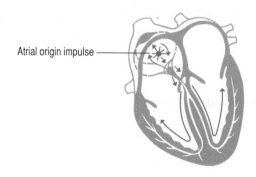

Atrial origin impulse

Because the atrial rate is slower in atrial flutter than in atrial fibrillation, the flutter (P) waves are easier to see on an ECG strip, and the ventricular rate is more regular. Atrial flutter typically occurs in clients with ischemic heart disease or valvular disease.

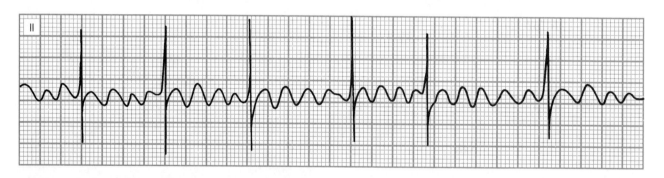

ECG characteristics

P wave   *Configuration:* The P waves, called flutter or F waves, appear in a sawtooth pattern.
Rate: The atrial rate may vary from 250 to 350 beats/minute, usually averaging 300 beats/minute.
Rhythm: The P-P interval is regular. Because a flutter wave is usually buried in a QRS complex, the arrhythmia can be overlooked by those monitoring the client. As the atrial rate nears 350 beats/minute, the rhythm may resemble a combination of atrial fibrillation and atrial flutter, called *atrial fib-flutter* or *flutteration*.

P-R interval   Usually, the P-R interval is not measurable; F waves outnumber QRS complexes, and determining which F wave was conducted to the ventricles proves difficult.

QRS complex   *Configuration:* The QRS complexes are usually normal and alike, but some may appear distorted if an F wave occurs simultaneously.
Rate: The ventricular rate can vary and is described in terms of AV conduction, or the ratio of F waves to QRS complexes (such as 2:1, 3:1, or 4:1). Usually, the ventricular rate will not exceed 200 beats/minute because of the AV node's inherent conduction speed.
Rhythm: The R-R interval may be regular or irregular.
Duration: QRS complex durations can be normal or, with an underlying intraventricular conduction defect, wide.

Effects on the client   With a diminishing of synchronous atrial and ventricular contraction comes a loss of atrial input (known as atrial kick) to cardiac output. This loss can reduce cardiac output by 10% to 30%. A client with limited cardiac reserve (for example, one with ischemic heart disease) may develop congestive heart failure. Atrial flutter also can produce rapid ventricular rates, further reducing cardiac output.

Treatment   Because atrial flutter is a transient, acute rhythm, synchronized cardioversion is indicated at initial doses of 50 to 100 watts/second. Atrial flutter caused by reentry also may respond favorably to overdrive cardiac pacing.
    Pharmacologic therapy may include:
- digoxin 0.25 mg I.V. or by mouth every 6 hours for four doses as a loading dose, then 0.25 mg daily. Decrease the dose if quinidine is to be added, because quinidine increases serum digoxin levels.
- quinidine sulfate 200 mg by mouth or intramuscularly every 3 to 4 hours or quinidine gluconate 324 mg every 6 to 8 hours. Quinidine, an antiarrhythmic drug that acts on the atria and the ventricles, also enhances conduction through the AV node; thus, digoxin should be administered before quinidine, because quinidine alone may increase the ability of the rapidly firing atria to conduct impulses to the ventricles, and ventricular rates may rise higher than 200 beats/minute.
- propranolol 10 to 40 mg by mouth four times daily or 1 mg I.V. every 5 minutes up to a maximum dosage of 3 mg.
- verapamil 80 mg by mouth three times daily or 5 to 10 mg I.V.; may repeat 10 mg I.V. in 30 minutes.
- procainamide (Pronestyl) 50 mg/minute by I.V. bolus until the arrhythmia subsides, the QRS complex widens by at least 50%, or the maximum dosage of 1 g has been administered; a continuous infusion of 1 to

4 mg/minute follows. The oral dose is 250 to 500 mg every 3 hours; that of the slow-release form (Procan SR), 500 mg to 1 g every 6 hours.

Nursing implications

- Because atrial flutter is commonly seen in clients with cardiac disease, ensure that the client is adequately oxygenated.
- The client is usually conscious before cardioversion; obtain an informed consent unless the client's condition prevents this.
- If the physician prescribes a short-acting sedative or an anesthetic, make sure that an anesthetist and resuscitative equipment are at the bedside.
- Ensure that cardioversion is not performed after digoxin administration; digoxin depresses the sinoatrial (SA) node, and cardioversion may cause bradycardia or asystole.

Practice example

Carefully study the ECG strip in the following example; then test your rhythm interpretation skills by filling in the blank lines with the appropriate information, using the knowledge you have obtained from this and earlier chapters. Check your responses against the correct answers provided later in this chapter on pages 86 and 87.

PRACTICE EXAMPLE

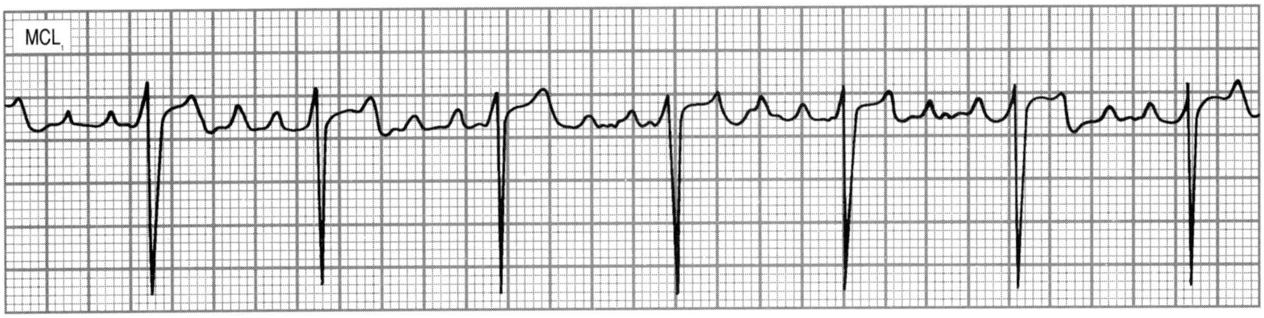

MCL

ECG characteristics

P wave   *Configuration:* _____

_____

Rate: _____

_____

Rhythm: _____

_____

P-R interval   _____

_____

QRS complex   *Configuration:* _____

_____

Rate: _____

_____

Rhythm: _____

_____

Duration: _____

_____

Interpretation   _____

_____

ATRIAL FIBRILLATION

In atrial fibrillation, many ectopic foci in the atrium fire rapidly at rates higher than 350 beats/minute. The impulse formation, which is similar to that seen in atrial flutter, occurs because of enhanced automaticity. The illustration below shows the sites of possible impulse formation. Arrows indicate the direction the impulse can travel.

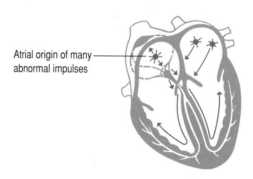

Atrial origin of many abnormal impulses

Because the AV node has a long refractory period, some impulses are blocked at the AV node when the atrial rate is higher than 180 to 200 beats/minute. When the AV node is no longer refractory, the ectopic atrial impulses are conducted to the ventricles at irregular intervals. Atrial fibrillation is associated with ischemic heart disease, mitral and tricuspid valvular disease, and chronic lung disease. It frequently occurs in clients after cardiac surgery and also is associated with hypokalemia.

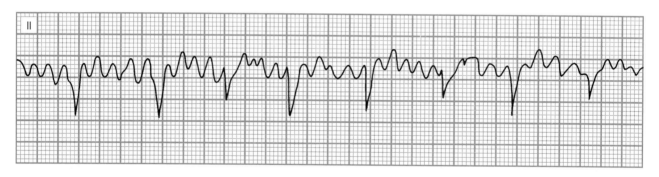

ECG characteristics

P wave   *Configuration:* Because the atria fire at rapid rates, P waves are not discernible; instead, a baseline of fibrillatory waves is seen. Difficult to identify at more rapid ventricular rates, these fibrillatory waves may be more visible when the R-R interval is longer.
Rate: The atrial rate is more than 350 beats/minute.
Rhythm: The atrial rhythm is chaotic and disorganized.

P-R interval No P waves are identifiable, so the P-R interval cannot be measured.

QRS complex *Configuration:* All QRS complexes should be normal and alike, unless aberrant conduction, an accessory pathway, or a ventricular conduction delay is involved.
Rate: The ventricular rate may vary. In uncontrolled atrial fibrillation, the heart rate exceeds 100 beats/minute and may rise as high as 180 to 200 beats/minute. Uncontrolled atrial fibrillation in a client with an unknown medical history usually signifies an untreated arrhythmia. In controlled atrial fibrillation, the heart rate is less than 100 beats/minute and usually signifies that the client is being treated with an atrial antiarrhythmic agent. An AV conduction block or digoxin toxicity should be suspected with slower rates. A complete AV block may be present if the R-R interval is regular, which indicates that none of the rapid atrial ectopic impulses are being conducted to the ventricles, causing the ventricles to beat independently. This rhythm is a classic sign of digoxin toxicity.
Rhythm: The R-R interval is completely irregular, with no pattern to the irregularity.
Duration: The QRS complex can be normal or wide, the latter signifying an underlying aberrant conduction, accessory pathway, or intraventricular conduction delay.

Effects on the client Atrial fibrillation causes a complete loss of synchronous atrial and ventricular contraction. This loss of atrial input (known as atrial kick) reduces cardiac output by 10% to 30%. In clients with limited cardiac reserve, such as those with ischemic heart disease, congestive heart failure may develop.

Treatment Atrial fibrillation usually is a chronic rhythm. Over time, thrombi may form on the walls of the quivering atria. Converting atrial fibrillation to a normal sinus rhythm with normal atrial contraction may loosen these thrombi and release them into the systemic or pulmonic circulation. Therefore, attempts to convert this rhythm to a normal sinus rhythm should be made only if the client's condition is acute and the medical record shows no history of atrial fibrillation. In such situations, synchronized cardioversion at 50 to 100 watts/second may successfully terminate the rhythm. After successful cardioversion, drug therapy may be used to prevent a recurrence. In chronic situations, the goal of therapy is to control the ventricular rate.

    Pharmacologic therapy may include:
- digoxin 0.25 mg I.V. or by mouth every 6 hours for four doses as a loading dose, then 0.25 mg daily. The drug should not be administered to clients who have digoxin toxicity. Decrease the dose if quinidine will be added, because quinidine increases serum digoxin levels.

- quinidine sulfate 200 mg by mouth or intramuscularly every 3 to 4 hours or quinidine gluconate 324 mg every 6 to 8 hours. Because quinidine enhances conduction through the AV node, digoxin must be started before quinidine is administered; quinidine alone may increase the ability of the rapidly firing atria to conduct impulses to the ventricles, causing ventricular rates to rise higher than 180 to 200 beats/minute.
- propranolol 10 to 40 mg by mouth four times daily or 1 mg I.V. every 5 minutes up to a maximum dosage of 3 mg.
- verapamil 80 mg by mouth three times daily or 5 to 10 mg I.V.; may repeat 10 mg I.V. in 30 minutes.
- procainamide (Pronestyl) 50 mg/minute by I.V. bolus until the arrhythmia subsides, the QRS complex widens by at least 50%, or the maximum dosage of 1 g has been administered; a continuous infusion of 1 to 4 mg/minute follows. The oral dose is 250 to 500 mg every 3 hours; that of the slow-release form (Procan SR), 500 mg to 1 g every 6 hours.

Nursing implications

- If the client is not on a cardiac monitor, suspect atrial fibrillation when the client's pulse is irregular and an apical-radial pulse reading reveals a pulse deficit.
- Assess the client for signs of congestive heart failure.
- Monitor serum digoxin levels, especially in atrial fibrillation with a slow ventricular rate.
- Never administer quinidine to a client in atrial fibrillation without first administering digoxin.
- Atrial fibrillation can have severe consequences when the client has an accessory pathway that bypasses the AV node. The accessory pathway usually has a refractory period shorter than that of the AV node, causing rapid ventricular rates that place the client at high risk for ventricular arrhythmias and sudden death.
- Digoxin is contraindicated in clients with a suspected accessory pathway because it prolongs the AV node refractory period, which enhances conduction of the impulse along the accessory pathway.

Practice example

Carefully study the ECG strip in the following example; then test your rhythm interpretation skills by filling in the blank lines with the appropriate information, using the knowledge you have obtained from this and earlier chapters. Check your responses against the correct answers provided later in this chapter on page 87.

PRACTICE EXAMPLE

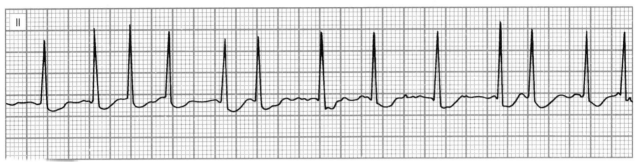

ECG characteristics

    P wave   *Configuration:* _____

                    _____

                    Rate: _____

                    _____

                    Rhythm: _____

                    _____

    P-R interval   _____

                    _____

    QRS complex   *Configuration:* _____

                    _____

                    Rate: _____

                    _____

                    Rhythm: _____

                    _____

                    Duration: _____

                    _____

Interpretation   _____

                    _____

WANDERING ATRIAL PACEMAKER

Wandering atrial pacemaker is caused by several different ectopic pacemaker sites in the atria and AV node, in addition to the SA pacemaker. These ectopic impulses are usually conducted normally through the AV node to the ventricles. A pacemaker site in the AV node, besides sending the impulse to the ventricles, also may transmit the impulse in a retrograde, or reverse, manner to the atria. The illustrations below show the sites of possible impulse formation. Arrows indicate the direction the impulse can travel.

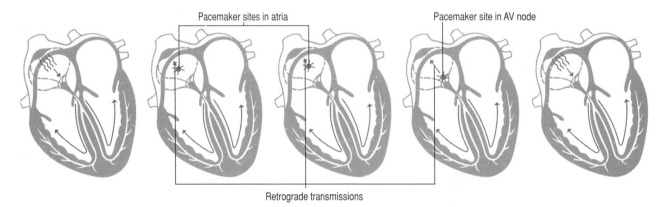

Pacemaker sites in atria

Pacemaker site in AV node

Retrograde transmissions

    This activity causes the P wave to appear inverted. Because some impulses do arise from the AV node or AV junction, the term *wandering atrial pacemaker* is not actually correct. The arrhythmia is associated with rheumatic heart disease, vagal stimulation, and digoxin toxicity.

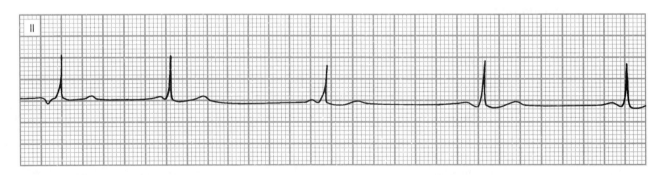

ECG characteristics

P wave *Configuration:* One P wave should precede each QRS complex. Because different pacemaker sites are involved, at least three different-looking P waves will be seen. This characteristic differentiates wandering atrial pacemaker from, for example, a normal sinus rhythm with a PAC, which may have two different-looking P waves. Some P waves may be inverted, which indicates an ectopic site in the AV node with retrograde conduction to the atria.

Rate: The atrial rate is usually 60 to 100 beats/minute but may be less than 60 beats/minute.

Rhythm: The P-P interval is irregular because of the different sites of impulse formation.

P-R interval

The P-R interval varies because of the different sites of impulse formation but remains within normal limits.

QRS complex

Configuration: All QRS complexes should be similar, and each QRS complex should be preceded by a P wave.

Rate: The ventricular rate is usually 60 to 100 beats/minute but may be less than 60 beats/minute.

Rhythm: The R-R interval is irregular because of the different sites of impulse formation.

Duration: The QRS complex is usually normal but may be wide if a coincidental intraventricular conduction defect exists.

Effects on the client

This rhythm usually produces no adverse hemodynamic effects unless the heart rate is slow enough to cause hypotension.

Treatment

No treatment is required unless the rhythm results from digoxin toxicity. In these cases, digoxin would be discontinued until therapeutic serum levels are reached. Atropine may be administered if symptomatic bradycardia occurs. Coughing may eradicate the rhythm by decreasing vagal stimulation.

Nursing implications

• Monitor the client for digoxin toxicity, bradycardia, and hypotension.
• This rhythm is usually benign and causes no adverse consequences.

Practice example

Carefully study the ECG strip in the following example; then test your rhythm interpretation skills by filling in the blank lines with the appropriate information, using the knowledge you have obtained from this and earlier chapters. Check your responses against the correct answers provided later in this chapter on page 87.

PRACTICE EXAMPLE

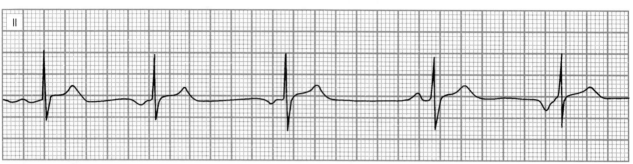

ECG characteristics

P wave   *Configuration:*

_____

_____

Rate:

_____

_____

Rhythm:

_____

_____

P-R interval

_____

_____

QRS complex   *Configuration:*

_____

_____

Rate:

_____

_____

Rhythm:

_____

_____

Duration:

_____

_____

Interpretation

_____

_____

MULTIFOCAL ATRIAL TACHYCARDIA

Multifocal atrial tachycardia, sometimes called chaotic atrial tachycardia, is characterized by its speed and by several P waves with different configurations. The impulses originate from various areas in the atria and are caused by enhanced automaticity. The illustrations below show the sites of possible impulse formation. Arrows indicate the direction the impulse can travel.

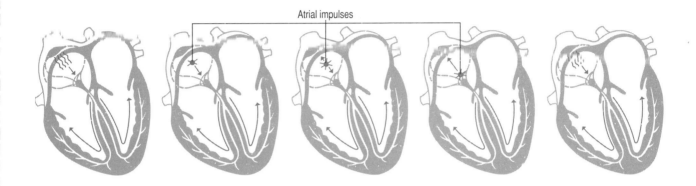

Atrial impulses

This rhythm commonly occurs in clients with chronic lung disease but also may develop in those with hypoxia, digoxin toxicity, or hypokalemia.

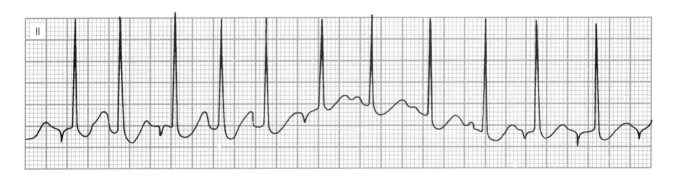

ECG characteristics

P wave *Configuration:* At least three P waves with different configurations are visible.
Rate: The atrial rate is 100 to 250 beats/minute.
Rhythm: The P-P intervals are irregular.

P-R interval The P-R interval varies but is usually within normal limits.

QRS complex *Configuration:* The QRS complexes should all appear similar.

Rate: The ventricular rate is between 100 and 250 beats/minute.
Rhythm: The R-R intervals are irregular.
Duration: The QRS complex is usually normal but may be wide if a coincidental intraventricular conduction defect or aberrant conduction is involved.

Effects on the client   The chaotic and rapid nature of this rhythm may reduce ventricular filling time and cardiac output.

Treatment   No satisfactory treatment exists, although a continuous infusion of verapamil I.V. at 5 mg/hour may help control the heart rate.

Nursing implications   • Assess the client's arterial blood gas values and serum potassium and digoxin levels.
• This rhythm is difficult to treat, and pharmacologic therapy may be ineffective.

Practice example   Carefully study the ECG strip in the following example; then test your rhythm interpretation skills by filling in the blank lines with the appropriate information, using the knowledge you have obtained from this and earlier chapters. Check your responses against the correct answers provided later in this chapter on page 88.

PRACTICE EXAMPLE

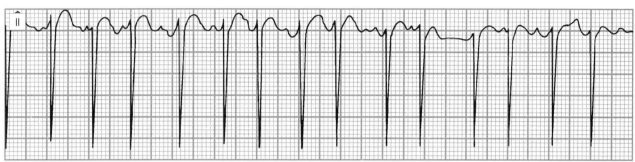

ECG characteristics

P wave   *Configuration:* _____

_____

Rate: _____

_____

Rhythm: _____

_____

P-R interval _____

_____

QRS complex   *Configuration:* _____

Rate: _____

Rhythm: _____

Duration: _____

_____

Interpretation _____

_____

ANSWERS TO PRACTICE EXAMPLES
PREMATURE ATRIAL CONTRACTION

ECG characteristics

P wave   *Configuration:* All upright and identical except for the 7th beat
Rate: About 95 beats/minute
Rhythm: Regular except for the 7th beat, which is premature

P-R interval   0.16 second for normal beats; 0.12 second for the 7th beat

QRS complex   *Configuration:* All normal and alike
Rate: About 95 beats/minute
Rhythm: Regular except for the 7th beat, which is premature
Duration: 0.10 second

Interpretation   Normal sinus rhythm with one PAC

PAROXYSMAL AND NONPAROXYSMAL ATRIAL TACHYCARDIA

ECG characteristics

P wave   *Configuration:* All upright and identical
Rate: 180 beats/minute
Rhythm: Regular

P-R interval   0.18 second

QRS complex   *Configuration:* All normal and alike
Rate: 180 beats/minute
Rhythm: Regular
Duration: 0.06 second

Interpretation   Atrial tachycardia

ATRIAL FLUTTER

ECG characteristics

P wave   *Configuration:* Sawtooth flutter waves are evident, with four flutter waves to each QRS complex
Rate: The atrial rate is about 300 beats/minute
Rhythm: The rhythm is regular but may appear irregular because one flutter wave is buried in each QRS complex

P-R interval   None measurable

QRS complex	*Configuration:* The QRS complexes are normal and alike; some appear distorted because of the simultaneous occurrence of flutter waves *Rate:* The ventricular rate is about 75 beats/minute *Rhythm:* The rhythm is regular *Duration:* The QRS complex duration is 0.08 second
Interpretation	Atrial flutter with 4:1 ventricular conduction

ATRIAL FIBRILLATION

ECG characteristics

P wave	*Configuration:* No discernible P waves, just a wavy baseline *Rate:* Not measurable *Rhythm:* Irregular
P-R interval	Not measurable
QRS complex	*Configuration:* All normal and alike *Rate:* About 130 beats/minute *Rhythm:* Irregular, with no pattern to the irregularity *Duration:* 0.08 second
Interpretation	Atrial fibrillation

WANDERING ATRIAL PACEMAKER

ECG characteristics

P wave	*Configuration:* Three different-looking P waves are visible, some upright, others inverted. One P wave precedes each QRS complex. *Rate:* About 50 beats/minute *Rhythm:* Irregular
P-R interval	Varies
QRS complex	*Configuration:* All normal and alike *Rate:* About 50 beats/minute *Rhythm:* Irregular *Duration:* 0.08 second
Interpretation	Wandering atrial pacemaker

MULTIFOCAL ATRIAL TACHYCARDIA

ECG characteristics

P wave   *Configuration:* Three different-looking P waves are seen
Rate: About 150 beats/minute
Rhythm: Irregular

P-R interval   Varies

QRS complex   *Configuration:* All normal and alike
Rate: Approximately 150 beats/minute
Rhythm: Irregular
Duration: 0.08 second

Interpretation   Multifocal atrial tachycardia

SELF – TESTS

You can verify your understanding of the material presented in this chapter by completing the following self-tests. Like the practice examples, the self-tests will assess your knowledge of ECG characteristics and rhythm interpretation. Additionally, they will measure what you know about treatments and nursing implications for each arrhythmia. Complete all four self-tests in this chapter before comparing your responses with the correct answers in Appendix A, pages 202 to 205.

SELF – TEST 1

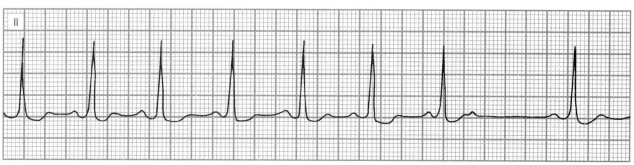

ECG characteristics

P wave *Configuration:*

Rate:

Rhythm:

P-R interval

QRS complex *Configuration:*

Rate:

Rhythm:

Duration:

Interpretation _____

_____

Treatment _____

_____

_____

_____

_____

_____

Nursing implications _____

_____

_____

SELF – TEST 2

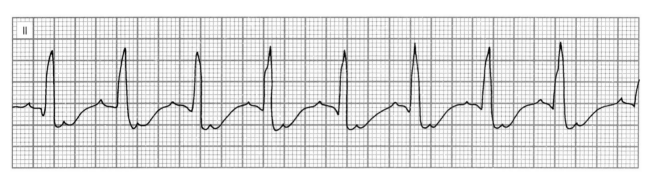

ECG characteristics

P wave   *Configuration:*
_____

_____

Rate:
_____

_____

Rhythm:
_____

_____

P-R interval
_____

_____

QRS complex   *Configuration:*
_____

_____

Rate:
_____

_____

Rhythm:
_____

_____

Duration:
_____

_____

Interpretation _____

_____

Treatment _____

_____

_____

_____

_____

_____

_____

Nursing implications _____

_____

_____

_____

_____

_____

_____

SELF – TEST 3

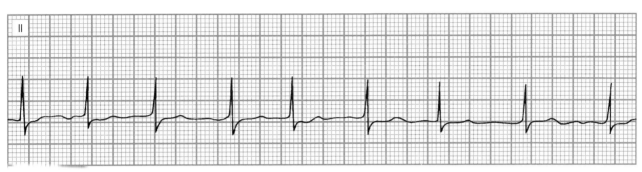

ECG characteristics

P wave   *Configuration:*

_____

Rate:

_____

Rhythm:

_____

P-R interval

_____

QRS complex   *Configuration:*

_____

Rate:

_____

Rhythm:

_____

Duration:

_____

Interpretation _____

_____

Treatment _____

_____

_____

_____

_____

_____

Nursing implications _____

_____

_____

_____

_____

_____

SELF – TEST 4

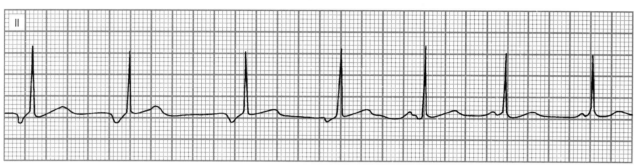

ECG characteristics

       P wave   *Configuration:*
_____

_____

                 Rate:
_____

_____

                 Rhythm:
_____

_____

   P-R interval
_____

_____

  QRS complex   *Configuration:*
_____

_____

                 Rate:
_____

_____

                 Rhythm:
_____

_____

                 Duration:
_____

_____

Interpretation _____

_____

Treatment _____

_____

_____

_____

_____

_____

Nursing implications _____

_____

_____

_____

_____

_____

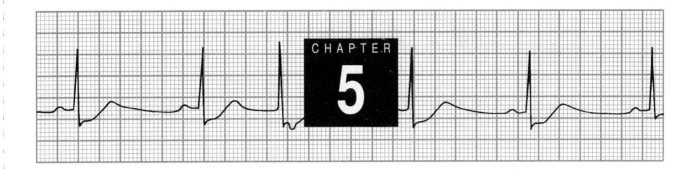

CHAPTER

5

Junctional Arrhythmias

Most junctional, or nodal, arrhythmias are associated with an escape mechanism or enhanced automaticity of the atrioventricular (AV) node or bundle of His. An escape mechanism occurs when the sinoatrial (SA) node fails to initiate an impulse, causing the AV junction (AV node and bundle of His) to take over as the dominant pacemaker. Escape mechanisms and enhanced automaticity commonly result from digoxin toxicity, a frequent cause of junctional arrhythmias. Some junctional tachycardias may result from reentry.

This chapter focuses on interpretation of the major junctional arrhythmias, including premature junctional contraction, junctional rhythm, accelerated junctional rhythm, and junctional tachycardia. For each rhythm, the text describes ECG characteristics, effects on the client, standard treatments, and implications for the nurse. To enhance learning, practice examples appear after the discussion of each arrhythmia, and the chapter concludes with three self-tests.

PREMATURE JUNCTIONAL CONTRACTION

A premature junctional contraction (PJC) is an ectopic impulse initiated early by the AV node or bundle of His and caused by enhanced automaticity of either site. The illustration below shows the site of impulse formation. Arrows indicate the direction the impulse can travel.

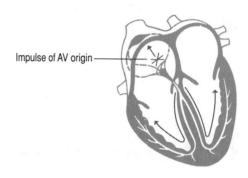

Impulse of AV origin

The impulse is conducted to the ventricles and may be conducted in a retrograde manner to the atria. PJCs are associated with digoxin toxicity, acute inferior myocardial infarction, rheumatic heart disease, valvular disease, and excessive caffeine intake.

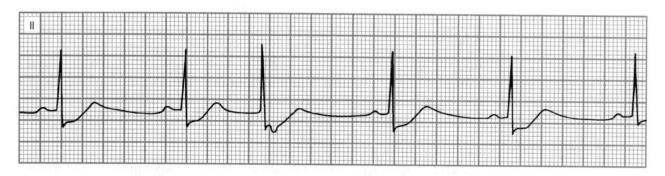

ECG characteristics

P wave   *Configuration:* The P waves may be absent, upright, or inverted in lead II and may occur shortly before or during the QRS complex or between the QRS complex and the T wave. The P waves' location depends on whether the atria or the ventricles receive the premature impulse first.
Rate: The atrial rate is the same as that of the underlying rhythm.
Rhythm: The P-P interval preceding the premature beat is shorter than the P-P intervals of the underlying rhythm.

P-R interval   If the P waves are upright and occur before the QRS complex, the P-R interval is less than 0.12 second. If the P wave is inverted or occurs during the QRS complex, the P-R interval is not measured.

QRS complex	*Configuration:* The QRS complex may be similar in configuration to the QRS complexes of the underlying rhythm. *Rate:* The ventricular rate is the same as that of the underlying rhythm. *Rhythm:* The R-R interval preceding the premature beat is shorter than the R-R intervals of the underlying rhythm. *Duration:* The QRS complex may be normal or wide; the latter indicates a preexisting ventricular conduction delay or aberrant ventricular conduction.
Effects on the client	PJCs are usually of little consequence, although the client may experience palpitations. Rarely, PJCs trigger reentrant junctional tachycardia.
Treatment	Treatment focuses on identifying and removing the cause (for instance, by withholding digoxin or restricting caffeine intake).
Nursing implications	• Monitor the client's serum digoxin level for signs of toxicity. • Encourage the client to reduce or eliminate caffeine intake if the PJCs are frequent or bothersome.
Practice example	Carefully study the ECG strip in the following example; then test your rhythm interpretation skills by filling in the blank lines with the appropriate information, using the knowledge you have obtained from this and earlier chapters. Check your responses against the correct answers provided later in this chapter on page 110.

PRACTICE EXAMPLE

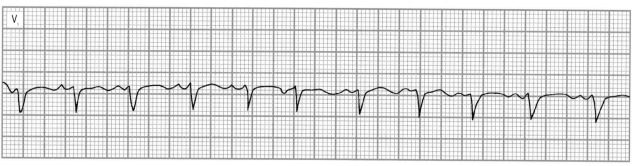

ECG characteristics

    P wave   *Configuration:* _____

_____

Rate: _____

_____

Rhythm: _____

_____

    P-R interval   _____

_____

    QRS complex   *Configuration:* _____

_____

Rate: _____

_____

Rhythm: _____

_____

Duration: _____

_____

Interpretation   _____

_____

JUNCTIONAL RHYTHM

Junctional rhythm is an escape rhythm, or safety mechanism, that occurs when the SA node fails to pace the heart. The impulse is conducted in a pattern similar to that of a PJC (see page 98 for an illustration of impulse formation). Junctional rhythm can be caused by organic disease of the SA node (such as sick sinus syndrome), acute inferior myocardial infarction, digoxin toxicity, rheumatic heart disease, or valvular disease. Clients in the immediate post-cardiac surgery period are particularly susceptible to junctional rhythm.

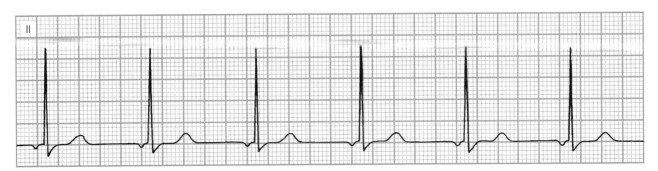

ECG characteristics

P wave *Configuration:* The P waves may be absent, upright, or inverted in lead II and may occur shortly before or during the QRS complex or between the QRS complex and the T wave. The P waves' location depends on whether the atria or the ventricles receive the impulse first.
Rate: If the P waves are visible, the atrial rate ranges from 40 to 60 beats/minute, the inherent rate of the AV node.
Rhythm: If the P waves are seen, the P-P interval is usually regular.

P-R interval If the P waves are upright and occur before the QRS complex, the P-R interval is less than 0.12 second. If the P wave is inverted or occurs during the QRS complex, the P-R interval is not measured.

QRS complex *Configuration:* The QRS complexes are usually normal and alike.
Rate: The ventricular rate ranges from 40 to 60 beats/minute, the inherent rate of the AV node.
Rhythm: The R-R interval is usually regular.
Duration: The QRS complex may be normal or wide; the latter indicates a preexisting bundle branch block or aberrant ventricular conduction.

Effects on the client A client may be able to tolerate junctional rhythm, especially if the heart rate is greater than 50 beats/minute. If the client cannot tolerate a low rate, cardiac output may drop, resulting in hypotension and decreased consciousness.

Treatment   The goal of treatment is to reestablish a sinus rhythm if the client experiences symptoms from the junctional rhythm. Possible treatments include administration of atropine (0.5 mg I.V. every 5 minutes up to 2 mg), a temporary pacemaker (for transient rhythms brought on by digoxin toxicity or acute inferior myocardial infarction), and a permanent pacemaker (for chronic rhythms).

Nursing implications   • Monitor the client's serum digoxin level for toxic elevation.
• Anticipate this rhythm in a client with an acute inferior myocardial infarction; a low heart rate may deprive the myocardium of oxygen and extend the ischemic area.
• Keep atropine and a temporary pacemaker at the client's bedside.

Practice example   Carefully study the ECG strip in the following example; then test your rhythm interpretation skills by filling in the blank lines with the appropriate information, using the knowledge you have obtained from this and earlier chapters. Check your responses against the correct answers provided later in this chapter on page 110.

PRACTICE EXAMPLE

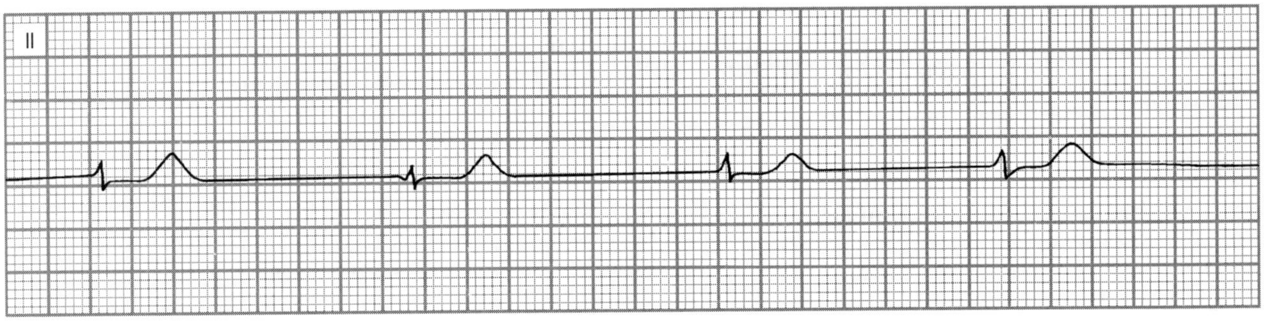

ECG characteristics

P wave   *Configuration:* _____

_____

Rate: _____

_____

Rhythm: _____

_____

P-R interval _____

_____

QRS complex   *Configuration:* _____

_____

Rate: _____

_____

Rhythm: _____

_____

Duration: _____

_____

Interpretation _____

_____

ACCELERATED JUNCTIONAL RHYTHM

Accelerated junctional rhythm is an ectopic rhythm caused by enhanced automaticity of the AV node or bundle of His. Impulse conduction is similar to that of a PJC (see page 98 for an illustration of impulse formation). Associated with digoxin toxicity or acute inferior myocardial infarction, accelerated junctional rhythm also can occur after infusion of a thrombolytic agent, such as streptokinase or tissue plasminogen activator, a condition known as reperfusion arrhythmia.

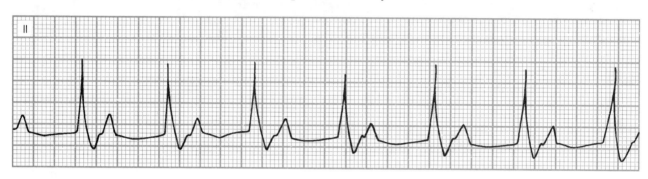

ECG characteristics

P wave *Configuration:* The P waves may be absent, upright, or inverted in lead II. They may occur shortly before or during the QRS complex or between the QRS complex and the T wave. The P waves' location depends on whether the atria or the ventricles receive the impulse first.
Rate: If P waves are seen, the atrial rate ranges from 60 to 100 beats/minute.
Rhythm: If P waves are seen, the P-P interval is usually regular.

P-R interval If the P waves are upright and occur before the QRS complex, the P-R interval is less than 0.12 second. If the P wave is inverted or occurs during the QRS complex, the P-R interval is not measured.

QRS complex *Configuration:* The QRS complexes are usually normal and alike.
Rate: The ventricular rate ranges from 60 to 100 beats/minute.
Rhythm: The R-R interval is usually regular.
Duration: The QRS complex may be normal or wide; the latter indicates a preexisting bundle branch block or aberrant ventricular conduction.

Effects on the client Most clients easily tolerate accelerated junctional rhythm because the heart rate is normal; the client's condition should be monitored closely, however, because this rhythm can deteriorate into a junctional rhythm.

Treatment No treatment is indicated unless the rhythm deteriorates into a junctional rhythm. If accelerated junctional rhythm occurs in a client with acute inferior myocardial infarction, administration of ventricular antiarrhythmic agents, such as lidocaine, should be discontinued: these agents can suppress the rhythm, thereby reducing the heart rate and possibly extending the ischemic area.

Nursing implications
- Monitor the client's serum digoxin level for toxic elevation, and discontinue the drug, if indicated.
- Anticipate this rhythm in a client with an acute inferior myocardial infarction.
- Keep atropine at the client's bedside in case the rhythm deteriorates.
- Consult with the physician on discontinuing infusions of ventricular antiarrhythmic agents.

Practice example
Carefully study the ECG strip in the following example; then test your rhythm interpretation skills by filling in the blank lines with the appropriate information, using the knowledge you have obtained from this and earlier chapters. Check your responses against the correct answers provided later in this chapter on pages 110 and 111.

PRACTICE EXAMPLE

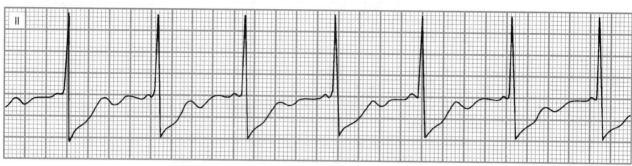

ECG characteristics

P wave   *Configuration:*

Rate:

Rhythm:

P-R interval

QRS complex   *Configuration:*

Rate:

Rhythm:

Duration:

Interpretation

JUNCTIONAL TACHYCARDIA

Junctional tachycardia is associated with enhanced automaticity of the AV junction or with reentry caused by a dual conduction pathway. In enhanced automaticity, the impulse is conducted in a manner similar to that of a PJC (see page 98 for an illustration of impulse formation). In reentry, the impulse returns to the AV nodal conduction system and reexcites conduction pathways that are past the refractory period. Junctional tachycardia associated with enhanced automaticity can result from digoxin toxicity or acute inferior myocardial infarction. Reentrant junctional tachycardia may be initiated by a premature atrial or junctional contraction. When the rate is greater than 180 beats/minute, this rhythm is difficult to distinguish from atrial tachycardia and may be referred to as supraventricular tachycardia.

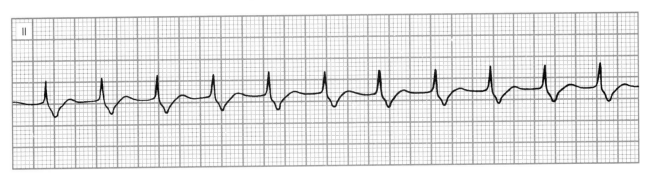

ECG characteristics

P wave *Configuration:* The P waves may be absent, upright, or inverted in lead II. They may occur shortly before or during the QRS complex or between the QRS complex and the T wave. The P waves' location depends on whether the atria or the ventricles receive the impulse first.
Rate: If P waves are seen, the atrial rate is greater than 100 beats/minute.
Rhythm: If P waves are seen, the P-P interval is usually regular.

P-R interval If the P waves are upright and occur before the QRS complex, the P-R interval is less than 0.12 second. If the P wave is inverted or occurs during the QRS complex, the P-R interval is not measured.

QRS complex *Configuration:* The QRS complexes are usually normal and alike.
Rate: The ventricular rate is greater than 100 beats/minute and can be as high as 180 to 200 beats/minute.
Rhythm: The R-R interval is usually regular.
Duration: The QRS complex may be normal or wide; the latter indicates a preexisting bundle branch block.

Effects on the client   If the heart rate is close to 100 beats/minute, the client usually can tolerate junctional tachycardia. This rhythm, however, can deteriorate into junctional rhythm if it is caused by digoxin toxicity. In such cases, digoxin should be discontinued. Reentrant junctional tachycardia is usually not well tolerated because it is more likely to occur at rates higher than 100 beats/minute. Clients with junctional tachycardia may exhibit signs of decreased cardiac output, such as hypotension, and decreased coronary perfusion, such as chest pain.

Treatment   No treatment is needed for junctional tachycardia caused by enhanced automaticity unless the rhythm deteriorates. If this rhythm occurs in a client with acute inferior myocardial infarction, administration of ventricular antiarrhythmic agents, such as lidocaine, should be discontinued, because these agents can suppress the rhythm, thereby reducing the heart rate and possibly extending the ischemic area. Vagal stimulation, synchronized cardioversion, or overdrive pacing may help control reentrant junctional tachycardia.

Pharmacologic therapy may include:
- verapamil 5 to 10 mg I.V.; may repeat 10 mg I.V. in 30 minutes.
- procainamide (Pronestyl) 50 mg/minute by I.V. bolus until the arrhythmia subsides, the QRS complex widens by at least 50%, or the maximum dosage of 1 g has been administered; a continuous infusion of 1 to 4 mg/minute follows.

If the reentrant rhythm is resistant to drug therapy, surgical ablation of the accessory pathway may be necessary.

Nursing implications
- Monitor the client's serum digoxin level for toxic elevation.
- Anticipate this rhythm in a client with an acute inferior myocardial infarction.
- Keep atropine at the client's bedside in case the rhythm deteriorates.
- Consult with the physician on discontinuing infusions of ventricular antiarrhythmic agents.
- Study the client's ECG strips to determine what initiated this arrhythmia. Suspect reentry if you note a premature atrial or junctional contraction.

Practice example   Carefully study the ECG strip in the following example; then test your rhythm interpretation skills by filling in the blank lines with the appropriate information, using the knowledge you have obtained from this and earlier chapters. Check your responses against the correct answers provided later in this chapter on page 111.

PRACTICE EXAMPLE

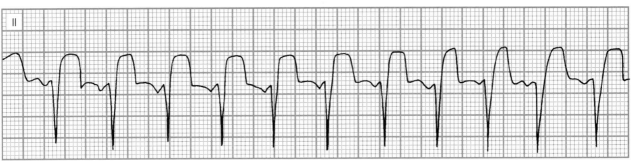

ECG characteristics

P wave   *Configuration:*

_____

Rate:

_____

Rhythm:

_____

P-R interval

_____

QRS complex   *Configuration:*

_____

Rate:

_____

Rhythm:

_____

Duration:

_____

Interpretation

_____

ANSWERS TO PRACTICE EXAMPLES

PREMATURE JUNCTIONAL CONTRACTION

ECG characteristics

P wave   *Configuration:* All upright and identical except for the 6th beat, which has an inverted P wave. One P wave is seen for each QRS complex.
Rate: 120 beats/minute
Rhythm: Regular except for the 6th beat, which is premature

P-R interval   0.18 second for normal beats; not measured for premature beats because the wave is inverted

QRS complex   *Configuration:* All normal and alike
Rate: 120 beats/minute
Rhythm: Regular except for the 6th beat, which is premature
Duration: 0.10 second

Interpretation   Sinus tachycardia with a premature junctional contraction (PJC)

JUNCTIONAL RHYTHM

ECG characteristics

P wave   *Configuration:* No P waves are visible
Rate: Not measurable
Rhythm: Not measurable

P-R interval   None

QRS complex   *Configuration:* All normal and alike
Rate: 40 beats/minute
Rhythm: Slightly irregular
Duration: 0.08 second

Interpretation   Junctional rhythm

ACCELERATED JUNCTIONAL RHYTHM

ECG characteristics

P wave   *Configuration:* All upright and alike
Rate: 69 beats/minute
Rhythm: Regular

P-R interval   0.10 second

QRS complex	*Configuration:* All normal and alike *Rate:* 69 beats/minute *Rhythm:* Regular *Duration:* 0.08 second

Interpretation   Accelerated junctional rhythm

JUNCTIONAL TACHYCARDIA

ECG characteristics

P wave   *Configuration:* Inverted P waves appear before the QRS complexes
Rate: 120 beats/minute
Rhythm: Regular

P-R interval   Not measurable

QRS complex   *Configuration:* All normal and alike
Rate: 120 beats/minute
Rhythm: Regular
Duration: 0.08 second

Interpretation   Junctional tachycardia

SELF – TESTS

You can verify your understanding of the material presented in this chapter by completing the following self-tests. Like the practice examples, the self-tests will assess your knowledge of ECG characteristics and rhythm interpretation. Additionally, they will measure what you know about treatments and nursing implications for each arrhythmia. Complete all three self-tests in this chapter before comparing your responses with the correct answers in Appendix A, pages 205 and 206.

SELF – TEST 1

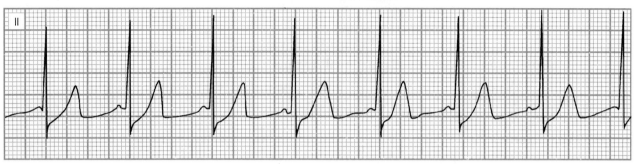

ECG characteristics

P wave   *Configuration:*

_____

_____

Rate:

_____

_____

Rhythm:

_____

_____

P-R interval

_____

_____

QRS complex   *Configuration:*

_____

_____

Rate:

_____

_____

Rhythm:

_____

_____

Duration:

_____

_____

Interpretation _____
_____

Treatment _____
_____
_____
_____
_____
_____

Nursing implications _____
_____
_____
_____
_____
_____

SELF – TEST 2

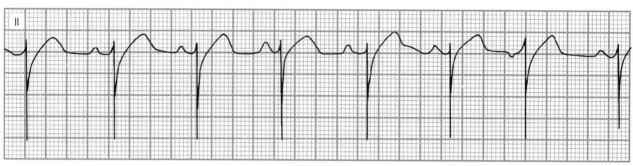

ECG characteristics

P wave   *Configuration:*

_____

Rate:

_____

Rhythm:

_____

P-R interval

_____

QRS complex   *Configuration:*

_____

Rate:

_____

Rhythm:

_____

Duration:

_____

Interpretation _____
_____

Treatment _____
_____
_____
_____
_____
_____

Nursing implications _____
_____
_____
_____
_____
_____

SELF – TEST 3

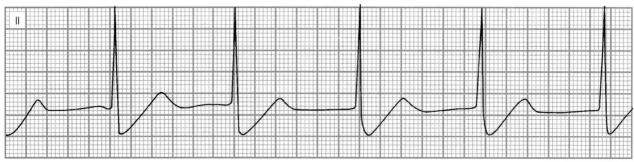

ECG characteristics

P wave *Configuration:*

_____

Rate:

_____

Rhythm:

_____

P-R interval

_____

QRS complex *Configuration:*

_____

Rate:

_____

Rhythm:

_____

Duration:

_____

Interpretation _____

_____

Treatment _____

_____

_____

_____

_____

_____

Nursing implications _____

_____

_____

_____

_____

_____

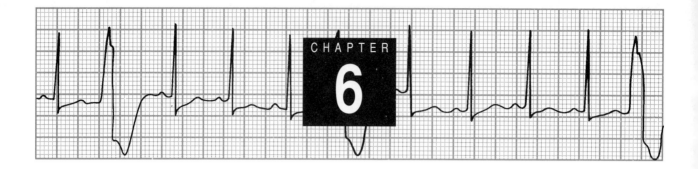

Ventricular Arrhythmias

Among the most common arrhythmias to develop in acutely ill clients, ventricular arrhythmias can be benign or lethal. In explaining how to discern a benign arrhythmia from a lethal one, this chapter focuses on interpretation of the major ventricular arrhythmias, including premature ventricular contractions, ventricular tachycardia, ventricular fibrillation, idioventricular rhythm, accelerated idioventricular rhythm, and asystole. For each rhythm, the text describes ECG characteristics, effects on the client, standard treatments, and implications for the nurse. To enhance learning, practice examples appear after the discussion of each arrhythmia, and the chapter concludes with four self-tests.

PREMATURE VENTRICULAR CONTRACTION

Premature ventricular contractions (PVCs) are ectopic impulses that originate in the ventricles; they are usually conducted in a retrograde manner through the nodal and atrial tissue.

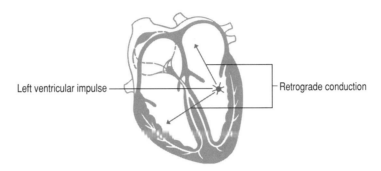

Left ventricular impulse —   — Retrograde conduction

Associated with enhanced automaticity of ventricular tissue or with reentry of a previous impulse, PVCs can be caused by digoxin toxicity, hypokalemia, caffeine, nicotine, stress, fatigue, mitral valve prolapse, sympathomimetic drugs, or myocardial irritability (from ischemia, hypoxia, pacemaker electrodes, or overdistended myocardial tissue). Clinical situations that commonly result in myocardial irritability include acute myocardial infarction, cardiac surgery, cardiomyopathy, and ventricular aneurysm. PVCs also can occur in healthy individuals; these rhythms are considered benign.

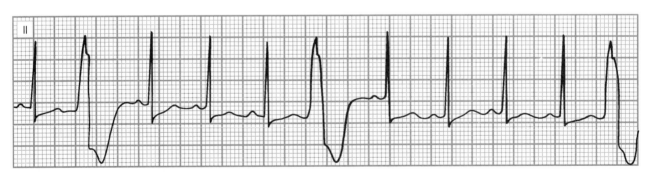

ECG characteristics

P wave *Configuration:* The P waves are similar to those of the client's underlying rhythm. They may be absent or, with retrograde conduction to the atria, may appear after the QRS complex.
Rate: The atrial rate is similar to that of the underlying rhythm.
Rhythm: The P-P interval will be regular or irregular, depending on the underlying rhythm.

P-R interval   The P-R interval is similar to that of the underlying rhythm.

QRS complex   *Configuration:* The QRS complex of a PVC is wide and bizarre in appearance. The T wave, for instance, may occur in the opposite direction from the QRS complex. If more than one PVC is visible and all are identical, they are called *uniform*; different-looking PVCs are called *multiform*. (Although the terms *unifocal* and *multifocal* are sometimes used, they are imprecise because they presume the same or different irritable foci; actually, the sites of irritability are impossible to determine by cardiac monitoring.)
Rate: The ventricular rate varies according to the underlying rhythm.
Rhythm: The rhythm may be regular except for the appearance of the early beat. PVCs occur earlier than normal beats, thus offsetting the rhythm's regularity. A PVC is usually followed by a compensatory pause; that is, the underlying rhythm does not reset itself, and the next normal beat does not occur when expected. An interpolated PVC is one that occurs between two normal beats without a compensatory pause. Other variations include ventricular bigeminy (every other beat is a PVC), ventricular trigeminy (one PVC for every two sinus beats or two PVCs for every sinus beat), and ventricular quadrigeminy (one PVC for every three sinus beats or three PVCs for every sinus beat).
Duration: The QRS complex duration is greater than 0.12 second because one ventricle is electrically activated before the other.

Effects on the client   Because PVCs produce abnormal conduction, inadequate cardiac output usually results; frequent PVCs can significantly diminish output. Additionally, PVCs can trigger more serious ventricular arrhythmias; for example, PVCs that occur during a myocardial infarction or that land on the T wave of the preceding beat (called R-on-T phenomenon) may precipitate ventricular tachycardia or ventricular fibrillation. PVCs are considered more ominous if they are multiform, occur in pairs, land on the preceding T wave, or occur more frequently than six times per minute.

Treatment   In the acute care setting, PVCs are treated with an intravenous antiarrhythmic agent. Pharmacologic therapy may include:
- lidocaine 1 mg/kg at a rate of 50 mg/minute by I.V. bolus followed by additional bolus doses of 0.5 mg/kg every 5 minutes until a maximum dosage of 3 mg/kg has been administered; a continuous infusion of 2 to 4 mg/minute follows.
- procainamide 50 mg/minute by I.V. bolus until the arrhythmia subsides, the QRS complex widens by at least 50%, or the maximum initial dosage of 1 g has been administered; a continuous infusion of 1 to 4 mg/minute follows (procainamide is administered if lidocaine proves ineffective or the client is allergic to it).

•bretylium 5 to 10 mg/kg, followed by a continuous infusion of 1 to 2 mg/minute (bretylium is administered if both lidocaine and procainamide prove ineffective).

   An oral agent (such as procainamide, quinidine sulfate, phenytoin, amiodarone, mexiletine, or disopyramide) is used for long-term treatment of PVCs.

Nursing implications
•If PVCs occur during an acute myocardial infarction, administer lidocaine as prescribed or according to institutional policy.
•Monitor serum digoxin and potassium levels and arterial blood gas values.
•Administer supplemental oxygen if prescribed.
•When treating PVCs with intravenous antiarrhythmic agents, place the client on a cardiac monitor and use an infusion pump for continuous infusions.
•Benign PVCs in a healthy individual may be a source of concern because they are associated with palpitations. The palpitations result from an increase in stroke volume that accompanies the next sinus beat after the PVC.

Practice example
Carefully study the ECG strip in the following example; then test your rhythm interpretation skills by filling in the blank lines with the appropriate information, using the knowledge you have obtained from this and earlier chapters. Check your responses against the correct answers provided later in this chapter on page 142.

PRACTICE EXAMPLE

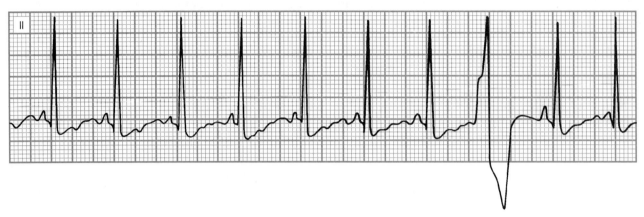

ECG characteristics

P wave *Configuration:*

_____

Rate:

_____

Rhythm:

_____

P-R interval

_____

QRS complex *Configuration:*

_____

Rate:

_____

Rhythm:

_____

Duration:

_____

Interpretation

VENTRICULAR TACHYCARDIA

Ventricular tachycardia originates in the ventricles in much the same way as PVCs, either through enhanced automaticity or, more commonly, through reentry of a previous impulse. A reentrant impulse can be initiated by a PVC that lands on the T wave of the preceding beat during the vulnerable relative refractory period (R-on-T phenomenon). Ventricular tachycardia can be caused by myocardial irritability from ischemia associated with acute myocardial infarction, congestive heart failure, or coronary artery disease, as well as from such cardiac conditions as ventricular aneurysm, cardiomyopathy, mitral valve prolapse, and rheumatic heart disease. Drugs that may precipitate ventricular tachycardia include digoxin; isoproterenol, which increases myocardial irritability; and quinidine, which prolongs the Q-T interval and lengthens the relative refractory period. Metabolic acidosis and hypokalemia also can cause ventricular tachycardia.

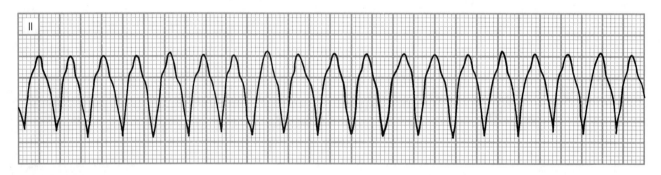

ECG characteristics

P wave
Configuration: The P waves are not usually visible but may occur after the QRS complex if retrograde conduction develops.
Rate: Not measurable
Rhythm: Not measurable

P-R interval
Not measurable

QRS complex
Configuration: The QRS complexes are wide and bizarre.
Rate: The ventricular rate is greater than 100 beats/minute.
Rhythm: The ventricular rhythm is usually regular.
Duration: The QRS complexes have a duration of more than 0.12 second.

Effects on the client
A client may be conscious and hemodynamically stable, unconscious and hypotensive, or pulseless and in cardiac arrest. Young clients and those without cardiac disease may tolerate the rhythm for a few hours; in other clients, the rhythm may deteriorate into ventricular fibrillation within minutes.

Treatment Therapy depends on the client's condition. Clients who have brief episodes of ventricular tachycardia are treated with an intravenous antiarrhythmic agent. A clinician who witnesses an episode of ventricular tachycardia may administer a precordial thump to terminate the arrhythmia through mechanical cardioversion.

Conscious and stable client This client should receive intravenous antiarrhythmic agents. Pharmacologic therapy may include:
- lidocaine 1 mg/kg at a rate of 50 mg/minute by I.V. bolus followed by additional bolus doses of 0.5 mg/kg every 5 minutes until a maximum dosage of 3 mg/kg has been administered; a continuous infusion of 2 to 4 mg/minute follows.
- procainamide 50 mg/minute by I.V. bolus until the arrhythmia subsides, the QRS complex widens by at least 50%, or the maximum dosage of 1 g has been administered; a continuous infusion of 1 to 4 mg/minute follows (procainamide is administered if lidocaine proves ineffective or the client is allergic to it).
- bretylium 5 to 10 mg/kg, followed by a continuous infusion of 1 to 2 mg/minute (bretylium is administered if both lidocaine and procainamide prove ineffective).

If antiarrhythmic drugs are unsuccessful, synchronized cardioversion at 50 to 100 watts/second may be needed. Synchronized cardioversion is timed with the client's heart rhythm so that electrical stimulation is not delivered during the T wave, or vulnerable period. This prevents the rhythm from deteriorating into ventricular fibrillation. The procedure can be repeated, if necessary, at 200, 200 to 300, and 360 watts/second. A conscious client should be sedated before undergoing cardioversion.

Unconscious or unstable client This client should receive synchronized or unsynchronized cardioversion (defibrillation), followed by antiarrhythmic agents. In defibrillation, the electrical stimulus is not timed to the client's intrinsic rhythm. This procedure is used only for potentially lethal arrhythmias, such as unstable ventricular tachycardia and ventricular fibrillation.

Pulseless client This client should receive defibrillation at 200 watts/second, increased to 200 to 300 and 360 watts/second until the arrhythmia subsides. Cardiopulmonary resuscitation should be performed between defibrillation attempts and antiarrhythmic agents administered. Epinephrine 0.5 to 1 mg should be given every 5 minutes followed by defibrillation at the maximum of 360 watts/second until the arrhythmia is terminated. The oral agents used for long-term treatment of ventricular tachycardia are the same as those used for long-term therapy of PVCs. If ventricular tachycardia recurs and does not respond to medical treatment, surgical ablation of the irritable foci may be necessary.

Nursing implications

- Know the hospital's policy; some hospitals have standing order protocols for specially prepared nurses to administer lidocaine and defibrillation, if necessary, until a physician arrives.
- Assess the client for acid-base or electrolyte imbalances, and check the client's chart for medications that may precipitate ventricular tachycardia.

VT vs. SVT with aberration

Distinguishing between ventricular tachycardia and supraventricular tachycardia with aberration is sometimes difficult (see *Two views of ventricular tachycardia*). The term *supraventricular tachycardia with aberration* is used to describe atrial or junctional tachycardia that occurs with a wide QRS complex. The correct diagnosis cannot be made from the client's clinical condition; for example, a client with ventricular tachycardia will not necessarily appear more unstable than a client with SVT with aberration. Ventricular tachycardia can be tolerated for a few hours, especially in young, previously healthy persons. Conversely, a chronically ill client with a history of cardiac disease may quickly become hypotensive with the onset of supraventricular tachycardia.

Two views of ventricular tachycardia

The first ECG strip shows ventricular tachycardia with a monophasic R wave pattern. The second strip shows ventricular tachycardia with a left notch, or rabbit ear, taller than the right in lead V_1.

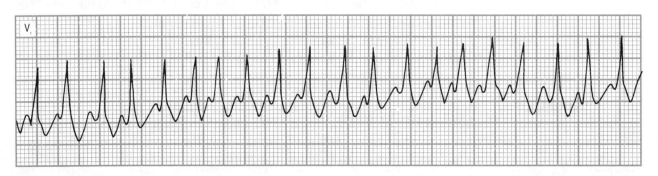

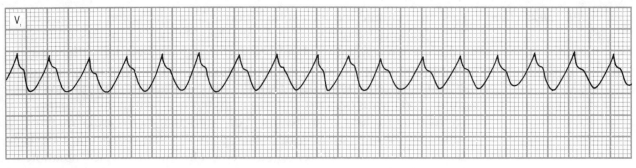

Factors that favor the diagnosis of ventricular tachycardia include:
- a QRS duration of more than 0.14 second
- a monophasic R wave pattern (a single, positive QRS complex) in lead V1 or lead MCL1
- a left notch (called a rabbit ear) taller than the right, if the QRS complex is positive in lead V1 or lead MCL1
- atrioventricular dissociation or asynchrony between the atria and the ventricles.

Factors that favor the diagnosis of supraventricular tachycardia with aberration include:
- a QRS duration of less than 0.14 second
- an rSR' pattern in lead V1 or lead MCL1 (a small R wave precedes the S wave; a larger R wave, called R prime, follows the S wave)
- an initial deflection of the QRS complex that is similar for both the normal and aberrant complexes, if rhythm strips of normal beats are available.

Supraventricular tachycardia

This ECG strip shows supraventricular tachycardia with an rSR' pattern in lead V1. The rhythm's QRS complex has the same initial deflection as that of the underlying rhythm.

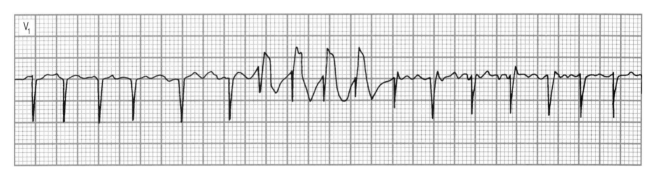

If the diagnosis remains uncertain, treat the client with procainamide, which has both atrial and ventricular antiarrhythmic properties. A client with ventricular tachycardia who is misdiagnosed as having supraventricular tachycardia may become hypotensive when treated with verapamil. Similarly, lidocaine may worsen the condition of a client with supraventricular tachycardia.

Practice example   Carefully study the ECG strip in the following example; then test your rhythm interpretation skills by filling in the blank lines with the appropriate information, using the knowledge you have obtained from this and earlier chapters. Check your responses against the correct answers provided later in this chapter on page 142.

PRACTICE EXAMPLE

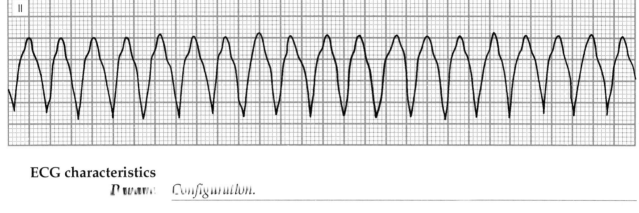

ECG characteristics

P wave   *Configuration:*

_____

Rate:

_____

Rhythm:

_____

P-R interval

_____

_____

QRS complex   *Configuration:*

_____

Rate:

_____

Rhythm:

_____

Duration:

_____

Interpretation

_____

_____

VENTRICULAR FIBRILLATION

Ventricular fibrillation is a chaotic, rapid rhythm that originates in the ventricles, usually as a result of a reentrant impulse. The illustrations below show two types of impulse formation in ventricular fibrillation. In enhanced automaticity, impulses can form at numerous sites. In reentry, the impulse follows a circular pathway.

ENHANCED AUTOMATICITY   **REENTRY**

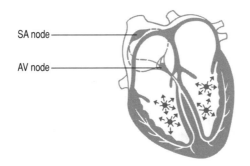
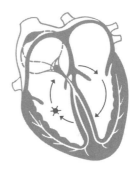

SA node

AV node

The chaotic rhythm causes the heart to lose its effectiveness as a pump, resulting in cardiac arrest. Ventricular fibrillation is caused by the same conditions that induce ventricular tachycardia; however, it also can occur spontaneously.

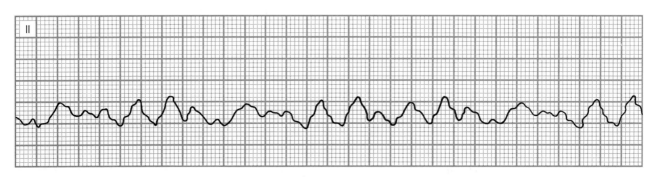

ECG characteristics

P wave   *Configuration:* The P waves cannot be identified.
Rate: Cannot be determined
Rhythm: Cannot be determined

P-R interval   Cannot be determined

QRS complex	*Configuration:* The QRS complexes cannot be identified. The rhythm is characterized by a wavy baseline. Large waves are described as coarse ventricular fibrillation; small waves, as fine ventricular fibrillation. *Rate:* The rate is rapid but cannot be determined. *Rhythm:* The rhythm is disorganized, chaotic, and completely irregular. *Duration:* Cannot be determined

Effects on the client No cardiac output is produced during ventricular fibrillation. The client will have no pulse and will be in cardiac arrest.

Treatment Coarse ventricular fibrillation is more easily terminated than fine ventricular fibrillation. A clinician who witnesses an episode of ventricular fibrillation may administer a precordial thump to terminate the arrhythmia through mechanical cardioversion. Defibrillation is begun at 200 watts/second and increased to 200 to 300 and 360 watts/second until the arrhythmia subsides. Cardiopulmonary resuscitation should be performed between defibrillation attempts and antiarrhythmic agents administered. Epinephrine 0.5 to 1 mg should be given every 5 minutes, followed by defibrillation at the maximum of 360 watts/second until the arrhythmia is terminated.

Long-term therapy for ventricular fibrillation is similar to that for ventricular tachycardia. Arrhythmias that do not respond to pharmacologic therapy may be treated by surgically implanting an automatic internal cardiovertor defibrillator (AICD), which recognizes ventricular fibrillation and defibrillates the heart internally.

Nursing implications
- Rapid recognition of the arrhythmia and rapid defibrillation are critical to successful treatment.
- Know the hospital's policy; some hospitals have standing order protocols for specially prepared nurses to administer lidocaine and defibrillation, if necessary, until a physician arrives. Support the airway by administering 100% oxygen during these procedures.
- Assess the client for acid-base or electrolyte imbalances, and check the client's chart for medications that may precipitate ventricular tachycardia.

Practice example Carefully study the ECG strip in the following example; then test your rhythm interpretation skills by filling in the blank lines with the appropriate information, using the knowledge you have obtained from this and earlier chapters. Check your responses against the correct answers provided later in this chapter on pages 142 and 143.

PRACTICE EXAMPLE

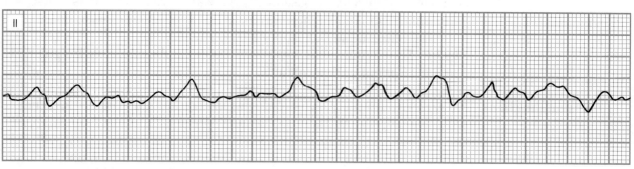

ECG characteristics

P wave   *Configuration:* _____

_____

Rate: _____

_____

Rhythm: _____

_____

P-R interval   _____

_____

QRS complex   *Configuration:* _____

_____

Rate: _____

_____

Rhythm: _____

_____

Duration: _____

_____

Interpretation   _____

_____

IDIOVENTRICULAR RHYTHM

Although idioventricular rhythm originates from the ventricles in much the same way as PVCs, it is an escape rhythm, not a premature ectopic rhythm. It occurs when the sinoatrial node fails to fire and the atrioventricular node fails to function as an escape mechanism.

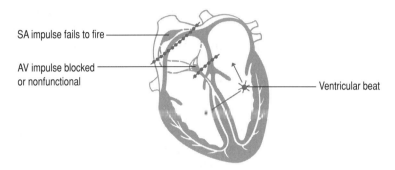

When these higher pacemakers do not function, isolated ventricular beats, called ventricular escape beats, occur. Idioventricular rhythm may develop in a client with a myocardial infarction, digoxin toxicity, or hyperkalemia.

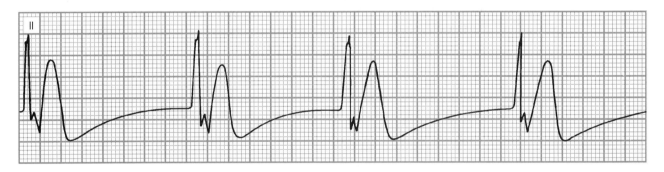

ECG characteristics

P wave   *Configuration:* The P waves are not usually visible but may appear after the QRS complex if retrograde conduction occurs.
Rate: Usually cannot be determined
Rhythm: Usually cannot be determined

P-R interval   Cannot be determined

QRS complex   *Configuration:* The QRS complexes are wide and bizarre.
Rate: The rate is between 20 and 40 beats/minute, the inherent ventricular rate.
Rhythm: The rhythm may be regular or irregular.
Duration: The QRS complexes have a duration of more than 0.12 second.

Effects on the client An idioventricular rhythm usually has serious hemodynamic consequences because of the slow heart rate it produces. Hypotension, loss of
consciousness, and seizures may occur.

Treatment The goal of treatment is not to eradicate the rhythm but to stimulate a
rhythm from a normal site in the conduction system. Atropine sulfate 0.5
mg I.V. every 5 minutes is administered until the maximum dosage of 2
mg is reached. A temporary pacemaker should be inserted or a transcutaneous pacemaker used. Isoproterenol 2 to 10 mcg/minute may be administered after the maximum dosage of atropine is reached and until a
pacemaker is inserted.

Nursing implications • Know the hospital's policy; standing orders may exist for a registered
nurse in a critical care unit or emergency department to treat this
rhythm with atropine until a physician arrives.
• Monitor the client's serum digoxin and potassium levels.
• Immediately discontinue any lidocaine infusions, because this drug depresses the conduction system.

Practice example Carefully study the ECG strip in the following example; then test your
rhythm interpretation skills by filling in the blank lines with the appropriate information, using the knowledge you have obtained from this and
earlier chapters. Check your responses against the correct answers
provided later in this chapter on page 143.

PRACTICE EXAMPLE

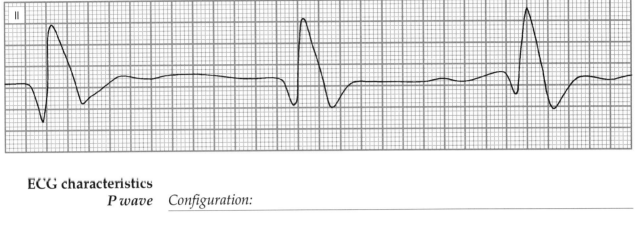

ECG characteristics

P wave *Configuration:* _____

_____

Rate: _____

_____

Rhythm: _____

_____

P-R interval _____

_____

QRS complex *Configuration:* _____

_____

Rate: _____

_____

Rhythm: _____

_____

Duration: _____

_____

Interpretation _____

_____

ACCELERATED IDIOVENTRICULAR RHYTHM

Accelerated idioventricular rhythm originates from the ventricles in the same way as idioventricular rhythm (see page 133 for an illustration of the impulse formation). The arrhythmia results from enhanced automaticity of an irritable ventricular foci, a common occurrence in acute inferior wall infarction. Accelerated idioventricular rhythm also can occur in healthy adults; in such cases, the rhythm is considered benign.

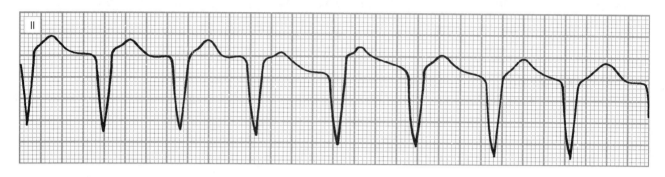

ECG characteristics

P wave   *Configuration:* The P waves are not usually visible but may appear after the QRS complex if retrograde conduction occurs.
Rate: Usually cannot be determined
Rhythm: Usually cannot be determined

P-R interval   Cannot be determined

QRS complex   *Configuration:* The QRS complexes are wide and bizarre.
Rate: The ventricular rate ranges from 40 to 100 beats/minute.
Rhythm: The rhythm is usually regular.
Duration: The QRS complexes have a duration of more than 0.12 second.

Effects on the client   This rhythm is usually well tolerated if the heart rate remains close to normal (60 to 100 beats/minute). Loss of atrial kick, however, may decrease cardiac output, and hypotension may develop.

Treatment   Treatment is not usually required because this rhythm produces a normal rate. However, if the rate drops to 40 to 50 beats/minute and hypotension develops, treatment similar to that for idioventricular rhythm may be needed.

Nursing implications   • Monitor the client for signs of decreased cardiac output, such as rales, tachycardia, and hypotension.
• Because accelerated idioventricular rhythm appears similar to ventricular tachycardia, question any administration of lidocaine, which de-

presses the conduction system. Lidocaine is unwarranted because this rhythm is usually benign.

Practice example   Carefully study the ECG strip in the following example; then test your rhythm interpretation skills by filling in the blank lines with the appropriate information, using the knowledge you have obtained from this and earlier chapters. Check your responses against the correct answers provided later in this chapter on page 143.

PRACTICE EXAMPLE

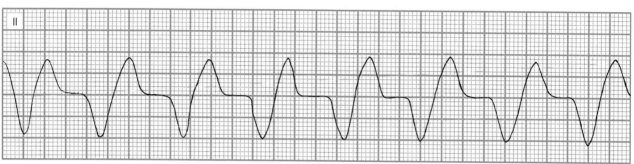

ECG characteristics

P wave   *Configuration:* _____

_____

Rate: _____

_____

Rhythm: _____

_____

P-R interval   _____

_____

QRS complex   *Configuration:* _____

_____

Rate: _____

_____

Rhythm: _____

_____

Duration: _____

_____

Interpretation   _____

_____

ASYSTOLE

Asystole, or ventricular standstill, is the absence of ventricular depolarizations. Atrial activity may or may not occur. A life-threatening arrhythmia that warrants immediate intervention, asystole can be caused by prolonged ventricular fibrillation, metabolic acidosis, hypoxia, or hyperkalemia.

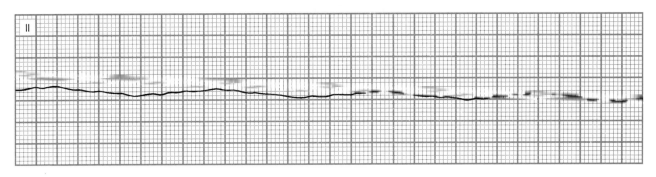

ECG characteristics

P wave *Configuration:* The P waves, which may or may not be visible, are not followed by QRS complexes.
Rate: Variable
Rhythm: Usually regular when it can be measured

P-R interval None

QRS complex *Configuration:* Asystole is usually characterized by a flat line. A wide QRS complex, called an agonal rhythm, occasionally occurs.
Rate: None
Rhythm: None
Duration: Not usually measured

Effects on the client No cardiac output is produced during asystole. The client will have no pulse and will be in cardiac arrest.

Treatment Cardiopulmonary resuscitation should be started immediately. Atropine 1 mg by I.V. push may be administered and repeated after 5 minutes. Epinephrine 0.5 to 1 mg I.V. is administered every 5 minutes. Transcutaneous pacing may be initiated or a transvenous pacemaker inserted. The client should be defibrillated in case the rhythm is actually fine ventricular fibrillation, which mimics asystole.

Nursing implications •Identify clients at risk for asystole (such as those with a myocardial infarction who develop an AV block or a bundle branch block) to prevent its occurrence; treatment for this rhythm is usually unsuccessful.

• During resuscitation attempts, monitor the client in more than one lead to rule out fine ventricular fibrillation.

Practice example   Carefully study the ECG strip in the following example; then test your rhythm interpretation skills by filling in the blank lines with the appropriate information, using the knowledge you have obtained from this and earlier chapters. Check your responses against the correct answers provided later in this chapter on pages 144.

PRACTICE EXAMPLE

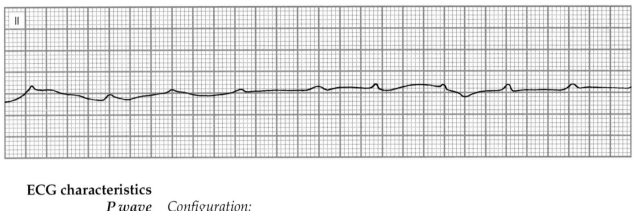

ECG characteristics

P wave   *Configuration:*

Rate:

Rhythm:

P-R interval

QRS complex   *Configuration:*

Rate:

Rhythm:

Duration:

Interpretation

ANSWERS TO PRACTICE EXAMPLES

PREMATURE VENTRICULAR CONTRACTION

ECG characteristics

P wave   *Configuration:* All normal and alike for normal beats but may occur after the QRS complex in abnormal beats. One P wave is seen for each QRS complex in the underlying rhythm.
Rate: 100 beats/minute
Rhythm: Regular except for the premature beat

P-R interval   0.12 second

QRS complex   *Configuration:* All normal and alike except for the premature beat, which is wide and bizarre
Rate: 100 beats/minute
Rhythm: Regular except for the premature beat
Duration: 0.08 second for normal beats; 0.34 second for the abnormal beat

Interpretation   Sinus tachycardia with one premature ventricular contraction

VENTRICULAR TACHYCARDIA

ECG characteristics

P wave   *Configuration:* Not visible
Rate: Not measurable
Rhythm: Not measurable

P-R interval   Not measurable

QRS complex   *Configuration:* Wide and bizarre
Rate: 210 beats/minute
Rhythm: Regular
Duration: 0.16 second

Interpretation   Ventricular tachycardia

VENTRICULAR FIBRILLATION

ECG characteristics

P wave   *Configuration:* Not visible
Rate: Cannot be determined
Rhythm: Cannot be determined

P-R interval   None

QRS complex   *Configuration:* Chaotic and disorganized, with a large, wavy baseline
Rate: Cannot be determined
Rhythm: Completely irregular
Duration: None

Interpretation   Coarse ventricular fibrillation

IDIOVENTRICULAR RHYTHM

ECG characteristics
P wave   *Configuration:* None visible
Rate: Cannot be determined
Rhythm: Cannot be determined

P-R interval   None

QRS complex   *Configuration:* Wide and bizarre
Rate: About 30 beats/minute
Rhythm: Irregular
Duration: 0.38 second

Interpretation   Idioventricular rhythm

ACCELERATED IDIOVENTRICULAR RHYTHM

ECG characteristics
P wave   *Configuration:* Not visible
Rate: Cannot be determined
Rhythm: Cannot be determined

P-R interval   None

QRS complex   *Configuration:* Wide and bizarre
Rate: 80 beats/minute
Rhythm: Regular
Duration: 0.24 second

Interpretation   Accelerated idioventricular rhythm

ASYSTOLE

ECG characteristics

P wave   *Configuration:* Visible but not followed by QRS complexes
Rate: 100 beats/minute
Rhythm: Regular

P-R interval   None

QRS complex   *Configuration:* None
Rate: None
Rhythm: None
Duration: None

Interpretation   Asystole

SELF – TESTS

You can verify your understanding of the material presented in this chapter by completing the following self-tests. Like the practice examples, the self-tests will assess your knowledge of ECG characteristics and rhythm interpretation. Additionally, they will measure what you know about treatments and nursing implications for each arrhythmia. Complete all four self-tests in this chapter before comparing your responses with the correct answers in Appendix A, pages 206 to 209.

SELF – TEST 1

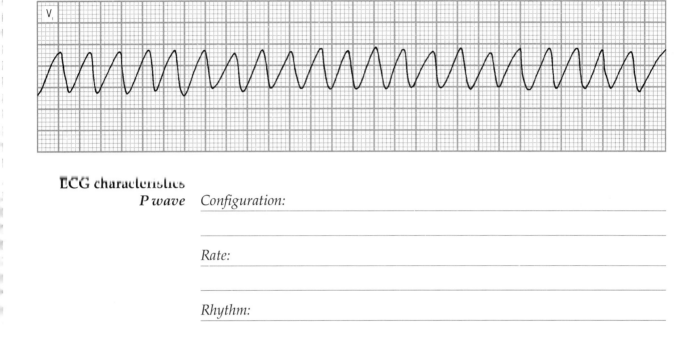

ECG characteristics

P wave   *Configuration:*
_____

Rate:
_____

Rhythm:
_____

_____

P-R interval
_____

_____

QRS complex   *Configuration:*
_____

Rate:
_____

Rhythm:
_____

Duration:
_____

Interpretation _____

_____

Treatment _____

_____

_____

_____

_____

_____

Nursing implications _____

_____

_____

_____

_____

_____

SELF – TEST 2

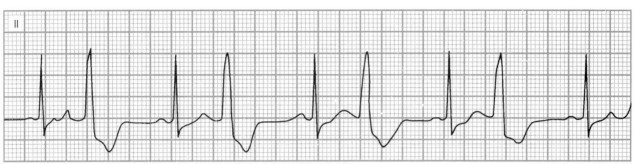

ECG characteristics

P wave   *Configuration:*

_____

Rate:

_____

Rhythm:

_____

P-R interval

_____

_____

QRS complex   *Configuration:*

_____

Rate:

_____

Rhythm:

_____

Duration:

_____

Interpretation _____
_____
_____

Treatment _____
_____
_____
_____
_____
_____
_____

Nursing implications _____
_____
_____
_____
_____
_____
_____
_____

SELF – TEST 3

ECG characteristics

P wave   *Configuration:*

Rate:

Rhythm:

P-R interval

QRS complex   *Configuration:*

Rate:

Rhythm:

Duration:

Interpretation _____

_____

Treatment _____

_____

_____

_____

_____

_____

Nursing implications _____

_____

_____

_____

_____

_____

SELF – TEST 4

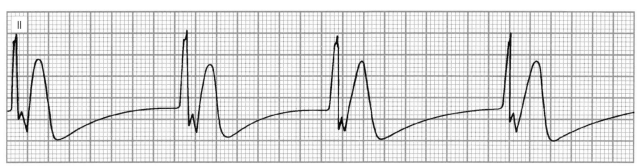

ECG characteristics

P wave *Configuration:*

Rate:

Rhythm:

P-R interval

QRS complex *Configuration:*

Rate:

Rhythm:

Duration:

Interpretation _____

_____

Treatment _____

_____

_____

_____

_____

_____

Nursing implications _____

_____

_____

_____

_____

_____

_____

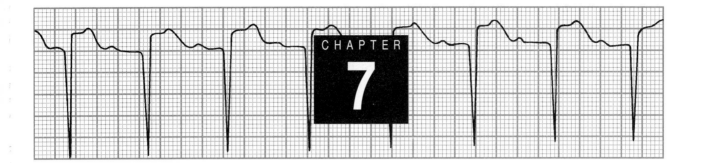

Atrioventricular Blocks

Atrioventricular (AV) blocks typically occur during a myocardial infarction because of the lack of blood flow to the AV node or bundle branches. This restricted blood flow results from ischemia or compression of the conduction system caused by edema associated with inflammation. AV blocks, which can be temporary or permanent, are most common in anterior and inferior infarctions. They are classified as partial (incomplete) or complete. First- and second-degree AV blocks are partial because some or all of the P waves are conducted to the ventricles. Third-degree AV blocks are complete because conduction at the AV node or bundle branches is completely interrupted. AV blocks can have minor or severe consequences, depending on the ventricular rate.

This chapter focuses on interpretation of the major AV blocks, including first-degree AV block, second-degree AV blocks (Mobitz types I and II), and third-degree AV block. For each rhythm, the text describes ECG characteristics, effects on the client, standard treatments, and implications for the nurse. To enhance learning, practice examples appear after the discussion of each arrhythmia, and the chapter concludes with four self-tests.

FIRST – DEGREE AV BLOCK

This arrhythmia is classified as a partial, or incomplete, block because the impulses, after originating in the sinoatrial (SA) node, travel down the conduction pathway and are slowed at the AV node, causing a prolonged P-R interval. The impulse then continues through the conduction pathway in a normal manner.

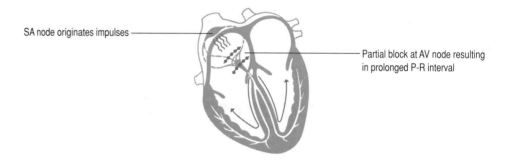

First-degree AV block is common in clients with digoxin toxicity, acute inferior myocardial infarction, degeneration of the conduction system, hyperkalemia, or rheumatic fever. The rhythm also occurs without sequelae in healthy persons.

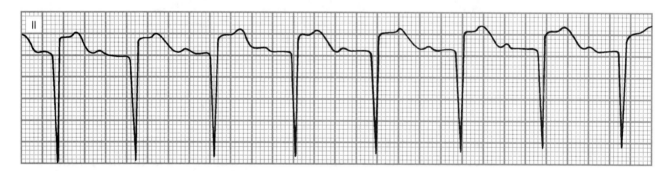

ECG characteristics

P wave *Configuration:* All P waves look normal and alike because the impulses originate in the SA node. One P wave is seen for each QRS complex.
Rate: The atrial rate is usually normal but may be abnormally slow, especially when the AV block is caused by conditions associated with bradycardia, such as digoxin toxicity or inferior myocardial infarction.
Rhythm: The P-P interval is usually regular.

P-R interval The P-R interval is longer than 0.20 second.

QRS complex *Configuration:* The QRS complexes are usually normal and alike.

Rate: The ventricular rate is usually normal but may be abnormally slow, especially when the AV block is caused by conditions associated with bradycardia, such as digoxin toxicity or inferior myocardial infarction.
Rhythm: The R-R interval is usually regular.
Duration: The QRS complex usually has a normal duration but may be wide with a preexisting ventricular conduction delay.

Effects on the client

The client usually tolerates this rhythm well unless bradycardia occurs. First-degree AV block can progress to second- or third-degree block, which have more severe hemodynamic consequences. This is especially likely in inferior wall myocardial infarction, during which transient AV blocks develop from edema formation at the AV node.

Treatment

First-degree AV block is usually not treated unless accompanied by bradycardia that results in hypotension and syncope. In such cases, atropine sulfate 0.5 mg I.V. every 5 minutes is administered until a maximum dosage of 2 mg is reached. A temporary pacemaker may then be necessary. After the maximum atropine dosage is delivered, isoproterenol can be infused at a rate of 2 to 10 mcg/minute if bradycardia persists and the pacemaker has not been inserted. However, isoproterenol increases the oxygen demand of the myocardial tissue, which may enlarge the ischemic area during an acute myocardial infarction.

Nursing implications

- Monitor the client's serum digoxin level, if indicated.
- Anticipate more serious degrees of AV block in clients with acute inferior myocardial infarction.
- Have atropine sulfate and a temporary pacemaker readily available.
- Administer supplemental oxygen, especially during an acute myocardial infarction.

Practice example

Carefully study the ECG strip in the following example; then test your rhythm interpretation skills by filling in the blank lines with the appropriate information, using the knowledge you have obtained from this and earlier chapters. Check your responses against the correct answers provided later in this chapter on page 166.

PRACTICE EXAMPLE

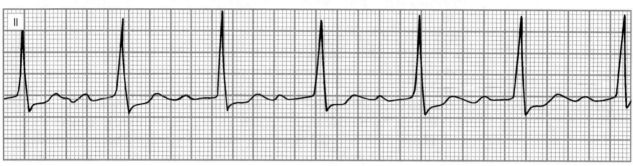

ECG characteristics

P wave *Configuration:* _____

_____

Rate: _____

_____

Rhythm: _____

_____

P-R interval _____

_____

QRS complex *Configuration:* _____

_____

Rate: _____

_____

Rhythm: _____

_____

Duration: _____

_____

Interpretation _____

_____

SECOND – DEGREE AV BLOCK, MOBITZ TYPE I

Second-degree AV block, Mobitz type I is a partial AV block. Impulses originate in the SA node but are progressively delayed at the AV node until, eventually, one impulse is not conducted to the ventricles.

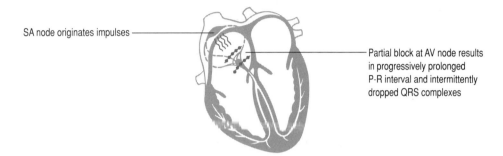

SA node originates impulses

Partial block at AV node results in progressively prolonged P-R interval and intermittently dropped QRS complexes

The pattern then repeats itself. Second-degree AV block, Mobitz type I is caused by the same conditions as those that cause first-degree AV block.

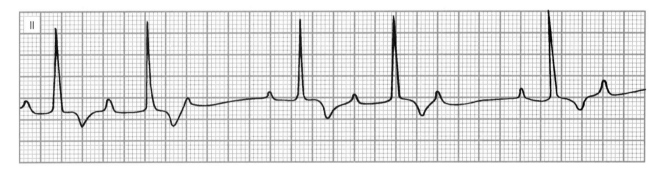

ECG characteristics

P wave   *Configuration:* All P waves look normal and alike because the impulses originate in the SA node. More P waves than QRS complexes are seen because the P waves begin to appear earlier and earlier in the refractory period until one occurs in the absolute refractory period, after which a dropped QRS complex is noted. The number of visible P waves in relation to the number of visible QRS complexes is described as a ratio (for example, 3:2 or 4:3).
Rate: The atrial rate varies according to the underlying rate of sinus impulse formation.
Rhythm: The P-P interval is regular.

P-R interval   The P-R interval becomes progressively longer until one P wave is not conducted to the ventricles, resulting in more P waves than QRS complexes. This event is called the Wenckebach phenomenon.

QRS complex	*Configuration:* QRS complexes are usually normal and alike, and each QRS complex is associated with a P wave.

Configuration: QRS complexes are usually normal and alike, and each QRS complex is associated with a P wave.
Rate: The ventricular rate varies but may be slow if many QRS complexes are dropped.
Rhythm: The R-R interval is irregular.
Duration: The QRS complex usually has a normal duration but may be wide with a preexisting ventricular conduction delay.

Effects on the client   Although considered more severe than first-degree AV block, second-degree AV block, Mobitz type I may be well tolerated. However, if the QRS complexes are frequently dropped, hypotension and syncope can result. This arrhythmia can progress to more serious AV blocks.

Treatment   No treatment is needed unless the client develops symptoms, such as hypotension and syncope. In such cases, treatment is similar to that for first-degree AV block. Atropine sulfate 0.5 mg I.V. is administered every 5 minutes until a maximum dosage of 2 mg is reached. A temporary pacemaker may then be necessary. After the maximum atropine dosage is delivered, isoproterenol can be infused at a rate of 2 to 10 mcg/minute if symptoms persist and the pacemaker has not been inserted. However, isoproterenol increases the oxygen demand of the myocardial tissue, which may enlarge the ischemic area during an acute myocardial infarction.

Nursing implications
- Monitor the client's serum digoxin level, and administer supplemental oxygen, as prescribed.
- Assess the client for hypotension.
- Have atropine and a temporary pacemaker readily available.

Practice example   Carefully study the ECG strip in the following example; then test your rhythm interpretation skills by filling in the blank lines with the appropriate information, using the knowledge you have obtained from this and earlier chapters. Check your responses against the correct answers provided later in this chapter on page 166.

PRACTICE EXAMPLE

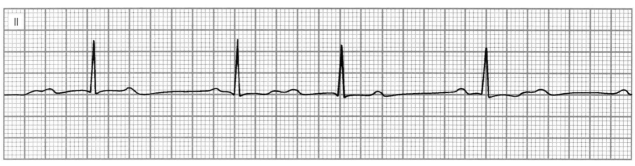

ECG characteristics

P wave *Configuration:* _____

_____

Rate: _____

_____

Rhythm: _____

_____

P-R interval _____

_____

QRS complex *Configuration:* _____

_____

Rate: _____

_____

Rhythm: _____

_____

Duration: _____

_____

Interpretation _____

_____

SECOND – DEGREE AV BLOCK, MOBITZ TYPE II

This arrhythmia is classified as a partial AV block. The impulse originates in the SA node but is then delayed and incompletely blocked at the bundle branches.

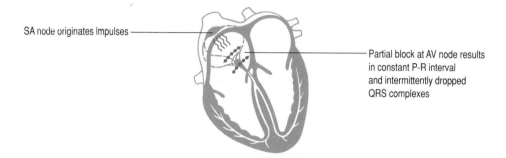

SA node originates Impulses

Partial block at AV node results in constant P-R interval and intermittently dropped QRS complexes

The QRS complex may be wide because the block occurs at the bundle branch level. Second-degree AV block, Mobitz type II is most commonly caused by an acute anterior wall myocardial infarction.

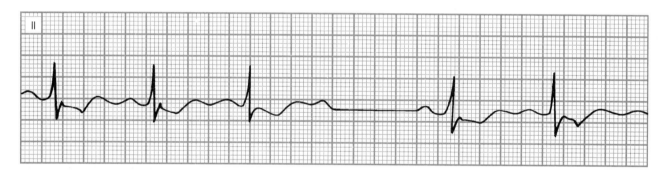

ECG characteristics

P wave   *Configuration:* All P waves look normal and alike because the impulses originate in the SA node. More P waves than QRS complexes appear.
Rate: The atrial rate varies according to the underlying rate of sinus impulse formation.
Rhythm: The P-P interval is regular.

P-R interval   The P-R interval, whether normal or prolonged, remains constant until a QRS complex is dropped. A rhythm in which every other QRS complex is dropped, resulting in a 2:1 ratio, commonly is characterized as Mobitz type II, although distinguishing between types I and II can be difficult.

QRS complex   *Configuration:* The QRS complexes may be wide and usually are all alike.
Rate: The ventricular rate may vary but usually is slow.

Rhythm: The R-R interval may be regular or irregular. A constant block ratio — for example, one in which every other QRS complex is dropped — results in a regular R-R interval. A variable block ratio results in an irregular R-R interval.
Duration: The QRS complexes may be wide.

Effects on the client

A Mobitz type II block is much more severe than a type I block. The rhythm is not well tolerated and results in hypotension and syncope. During an anterior wall myocardial infarction, this AV block is usually permanent because of the anoxic destruction of the conduction system in the bundle branches.

Treatment

Treatment is usually initiated immediately. The drug of choice is atropine sulfate 0.5 mg I.V. every 5 minutes until a maximum dosage of 2 mg is reached. A temporary pacemaker may then be necessary. After the maximum atropine dosage is delivered, isoproterenol can be infused at a rate of 2 to 10 mcg/minute if symptoms persist and the pacemaker has not been inserted. However, isoproterenol increases the oxygen demand of the myocardial tissue, which may enlarge the ischemic area during an acute myocardial infarction. In anterior wall myocardial infarction, a permanent pacemaker may be required.

Nursing implications

- Much more severe than lesser degrees of AV block, Mobitz type II usually constitutes an emergency.
- Immediately prepare the client for temporary pacemaker insertion, if needed.
- Have resuscitative equipment readily available.
- Administer oxygen as needed, and place a hypotensive client in a supine position.

Practice example

Carefully study the ECG strip in the following example; then test your rhythm interpretation skills by filling in the blank lines with the appropriate information, using the knowledge you have obtained from this and earlier chapters. Check your responses against the correct answers provided later in this chapter on pages 166 and 167.

PRACTICE EXAMPLE

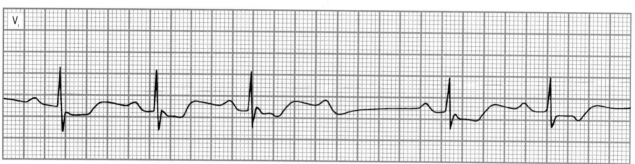

ECG characteristics

P wave   *Configuration:* _____

_____

Rate: _____

_____

Rhythm: _____

_____

P-R interval _____

_____

QRS complex   *Configuration:* _____

_____

Rate: _____

_____

Rhythm: _____

_____

Duration: _____

_____

Interpretation _____

_____

THIRD – DEGREE AV BLOCK

Third-degree AV block can be categorized under the general term *AV dissociation*, which means a lack of synchrony between the atria and the ventricles. In a third-degree AV block, the impulse originates in the SA node but is completely blocked at the AV node; an escape junctional or ventricular rhythm occurs to maintain ventricular contraction. Thus, in this rhythm, the atria and the ventricles beat independently.

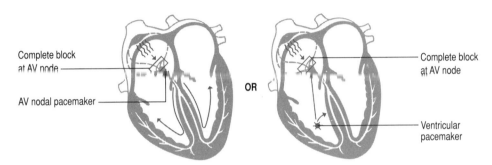

Third-degree AV block is caused by inferior myocardial infarction (especially infarction associated with right ventricular damage), anterior myocardial infarction, digoxin toxicity, mitral valve surgery, and rheumatic fever. It also can occur transiently during such procedures as angioplasty or cardiac catheterization.

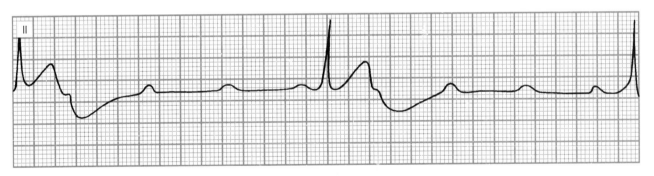

ECG characteristics

P wave   *Configuration:* The P waves are normal and alike.
Rate: The atrial rate may vary but is usually normal.
Rhythm: The P-P interval is regular, but some P waves may be masked by the simultaneous occurrence of QRS complexes. Additionally, the P waves may appear to march through the QRS complexes because they occur at a faster rate and do not relate to the QRS complexes.

P-R interval   No identifiable pattern emerges because the atria and the ventricles beat independently.

QRS complex *Configuration:* The QRS complexes may be normal (if the escape site is at the AV node) or wide (if the escape site is in the ventricles).
Rate: The ventricular rate reflects the inherent rate of the escape rhythm, which is usually slower than normal.
Rhythm: The R-R interval is usually regular.
Duration: The QRS complex may be normal or wide, depending on the site of the escape mechanism.

Effects on the client The slow heart rate induced by this rhythm usually results in hypotension and syncope.

Treatment Treatment is usually initiated immediately. Atropine sulfate 0.5 mg I.V. is administered every 5 minutes until a maximum dosage of 2 mg is reached. A temporary pacemaker may then be necessary. After the maximum atropine dosage is delivered, isoproterenol can be infused at a rate of 2 to 10 mcg/minute if symptoms persist and the pacemaker has not been inserted. However, isoproterenol increases the oxygen demand of the myocardial tissue, which may enlarge the ischemic area during an acute myocardial infarction. In anterior wall myocardial infarctions, a permanent pacemaker may be required.

Nursing implications
- Much more severe than either first-degree AV block or second-degree Mobitz type I, third-degree AV block usually constitutes an emergency.
- Immediately prepare the client for temporary pacemaker insertion, if needed.
- Have resuscitative equipment readily available.
- Administer oxygen as needed, and place a hypotensive client in a supine position.

Practice example Carefully study the ECG strip in the following example; then test your rhythm interpretation skills by filling in the blank lines with the appropriate information, using the knowledge you have obtained from this and earlier chapters. Check your responses against the correct answers provided later in this chapter on page 167.

PRACTICE EXAMPLE

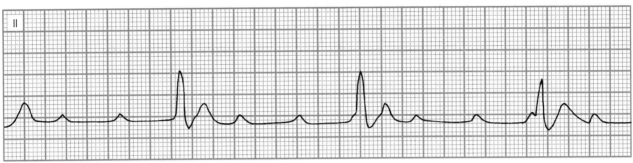

ECG characteristics

P wave   *Configuration:*

           Rate:

           Rhythm:

P-R interval

QRS complex   *Configuration:*

           Rate:

           Rhythm:

           Duration:

Interpretation

ANSWERS TO PRACTICE EXAMPLES
FIRST – DEGREE AV BLOCK

ECG characteristics

P wave   *Configuration:* All upright and identical; one P wave appears for each QRS complex
Rate: 63 beats/minute
Rhythm: Regular

P-R interval   0.40 second

QRS complex   *Configuration:* All wide and alike
Rate: 63 beats/minute
Rhythm: Regular
Duration: 0.12 second

Interpretation   First-degree AV block

SECOND – DEGREE AV BLOCK, MOBITZ TYPE I

ECG characteristics

P wave   *Configuration:* All upright and alike; more P waves than QRS complexes
Rate: 75 beats/minute
Rhythm: Regular

P-R interval   Varies from 0.24 second to 0.48 second

QRS complex   *Configuration:* All normal and alike
Rate: About 40 beats/minute
Rhythm: Irregular
Duration: 0.06 second

Interpretation   Second-degree AV block, Mobitz type I

SECOND – DEGREE AV BLOCK, MOBITZ TYPE II

ECG characteristics

P wave   *Configuration:* All upright and identical, with a 4:3 ratio of P waves to QRS complexes
Rate: 63 beats/minute
Rhythm: Regular

P-R interval   0.28 second

QRS complex   *Configuration:* All normal and alike
Rate: About 50 beats/minute
Rhythm: Regular except for dropped QRS complexes
Duration: 0.08 second

Interpretation   Second-degree AV block, Mobitz type II

THIRD – DEGREE AV BLOCK

ECG characteristics
P wave   *Configuration:* All upright and identical, with no identifiable ratio of P
waves to QRS complexes
Rate: 110 beats/minute
Rhythm: Regular; P waves march through QRS complexes

P-R interval   None

QRS complex   *Configuration:* All wide and alike
Rate: About 30 beats/minute
Rhythm: Regular
Duration: 0.12 second

Interpretation   Third-degree AV block

SELF – TESTS

You can verify your understanding of the material presented in this chapter by completing the following self-tests. Like the practice examples, the self-tests will assess your knowledge of ECG characteristics and rhythm interpretation. Additionally, they will measure what you know about treatments and nursing implications for each arrhythmia. Complete all four self-tests in this chapter before comparing your responses with the correct answers in Appendix A, pages 210 to 212.

SELF – TEST 1

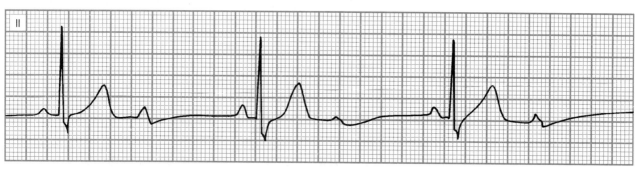

ECG characteristics

P wave   *Configuration:*

_____

Rate:

_____

Rhythm:

_____

P-R interval

_____

QRS complex   *Configuration:*

_____

Rate:

_____

Rhythm:

_____

Duration:

_____

Interpretation

Treatment

Nursing implications

SELF – TEST 2

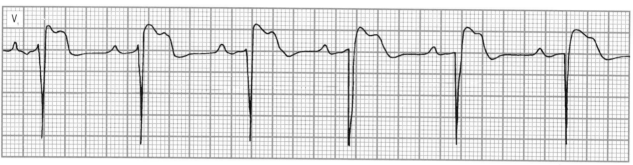

ECG characteristics

P wave Configuration:

_____

Rate:

_____

Rhythm:

_____

P-R interval

_____

_____

QRS complex Configuration:

_____

Rate:

_____

Rhythm:

_____

Duration:

_____

Interpretation _____
_____

Treatment _____
_____
_____
_____
_____
_____

Nursing implications _____
_____
_____
_____
_____
_____

SELF – TEST 3

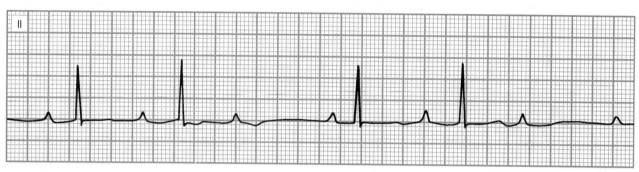

ECG characteristics

P wave   *Configuration:*

_____

_____

Rate:

_____

_____

Rhythm:

_____

_____

P-R interval

_____

_____

QRS complex   *Configuration:*

_____

_____

Rate:

_____

_____

Rhythm:

_____

_____

Duration:

_____

_____

Interpretation _____

_____

Treatment _____

_____

_____

_____

_____

_____

Nursing implications _____

_____

_____

_____

_____

_____

SELF – TEST 4

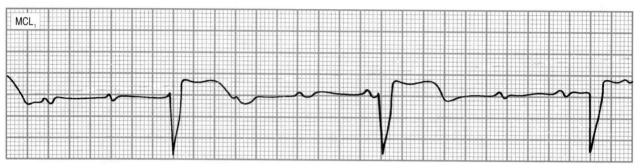

ECG characteristics

P wave   *Configuration:* _____

_____

Rate: _____

_____

Rhythm: _____

_____

P-R interval _____

_____

QRS complex   *Configuration:* _____

_____

Rate: _____

_____

Rhythm: _____

_____

Duration: _____

_____

Interpretation

_____

_____

Treatment

_____

_____

_____

_____

_____

_____

Nursing implications

_____

_____

_____

_____

_____

_____

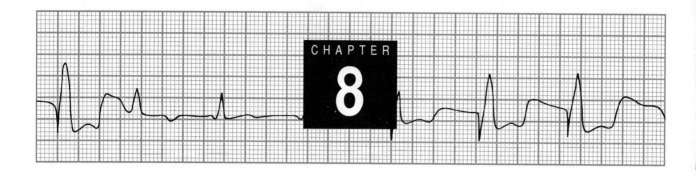

Pacemakers and Paced Rhythms

A pacemaker is usually needed when a client's slow heart rate reduces cardiac output, producing such symptoms as hypotension and syncope. Transient bradycardias, such as those caused by digoxin toxicity, may be treated with a temporary pacemaker until symptoms are reversed. Permanent damage to the conduction system, such as that which can occur from a myocardial infarction, may necessitate a permanent pacemaker. A pacemaker can stimulate the atrium or the ventricle or both. In addition, a pacemaker can sense a client's intrinsic rhythm and pace the heart only when the client's rate falls below a preset level.

This chapter describes indications for pacing, types of pacemakers, components of the pacemaker system, pacemaker classification codes, and common complications of pacing. Throughout, a systematic approach is provided for assessing properly paced rhythms. To enhance learning, the chapter concludes with a practice example and three self-tests.

INDICATIONS FOR PACING

A *temporary pacemaker* may be necessary in emergencies in which a client's heart rate is slow enough to decrease cardiac output. The pacemaker may be used to increase the heart rate (as in cardiac arrest; symptomatic sinus bradycardia; second-degree AV block, Mobitz type II; and complete heart block), to increase cardiac output and prevent cardiac arrest (as in open-heart surgery), to provide prophylactic therapy (as in cardiac catheterization), or to override tachyarrhythmias (as in overdrive pacing).

Reversible bradycardias and AV blocks commonly result when medications depress the conduction system or a myocardial infarction temporarily interrupts it. Digoxin is the most common conduction system depressant; other medications that can cause reversible bradycardias include phenytoin (an anticonvulsant) and thioridazine (an antidepressant). An inferior myocardial infarction can cause transient sinus bradycardia or AV block from edema formation near the conduction system. A temporary pacemaker may be inserted if hypotension develops from these arrhythmias, which can persist for several days.

Temporary pacing is accomplished transvenously, epicardially, or transcutaneously. A transvenous pacemaker is inserted into a large vein (usually the subclavian or internal jugular) and threaded into the right side of the heart. An epicardial pacemaker is attached to the outside of the heart wall and exits through the chest wall; this type is commonly used during open-heart surgery because the chest wall is already open. A transcutaneous pacemaker is attached to the chest wall with paddles, similar to those of a defibrillator; because it is easily attached, a transcutaneous pacemaker is commonly used early in an emergency until a transvenous pacemaker can be inserted.

A *permanent pacemaker* is inserted transvenously to increase heart rate and cardiac output in response to symptomatic and irreversible sinus bradycardia; sinus arrest; second-degree AV block, Mobitz type II; complete heart block; slow atrial fibrillation; bifascicular block; and sick sinus syndrome. Bifascicular block is a right bundle branch block that occurs with left anterior or posterior bundle branch block. Sick sinus syndrome is a degenerative process of the sinoatrial node that can produce sinus bradycardia, slow atrial fibrillation, or alternating periods of bradycardia and tachycardia. Any of these arrhythmias may occur during an acute myocardial infarction. Anterior wall myocardial infarction usually produces permanent AV blocks that result from permanent disruption of the conduction system. Degeneration of the conduction system (such as that seen in clients with rheumatic heart disease or Lenegre's disease) or surgical interruption of the system (such as during open-heart surgery or placement of intracardiac catheters) also can cause arrhythmias that necessitate a permanent pacemaker.

TYPES OF PACEMAKERS

The *demand,* or *synchronous,* pacemaker is synchronized with the client's normal, or intrinsic, rhythm; that is, the pulse generator fires only when the client's heart rate falls below a set rate. For example, if a demand pacemaker is set at a rate of 72 beats/minute, it would stimulate the heart to pace when the client's rate falls below 72 beats/minute. A demand pacemaker can be programmed to accommodate different heart rates. A rhythm strip of a demand pacemaker is shown below.

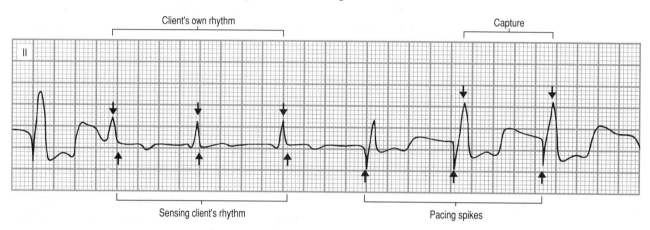

In this figure, the first and the last three QRS complexes are paced beats, initiated by a spike (the deep negative line seen before the QRS complex). The spike represents the pacemaker's electrical output. Capture (successful electrical stimulation of the myocardium) is indicated when the pacing spikes are followed by QRS complexes. The second, third, and fourth beats are the client's intrinsic rhythm. The pacemaker is inhibited when it senses the client's own rhythm, and it does not fire until the rate falls below 72 beats/minute.

The *fixed-rate,* or *asynchronous,* pacemaker fires at a constant rate regardless of the client's intrinsic rate and rhythm. Fixed-rate pacemakers were introduced in the 1950s and 1960s. Today this type of pacemaker is used primarily when the client has no intrinsic heart rate, such as during cardiac arrest. Most temporary pacemakers have a fixed-rate mode, and permanent pacemakers may convert to a fixed rate when a magnet is placed over the pulse generator. Because a fixed-rate pacemaker competes with the client's own heart rhythm, it can induce ventricular arrhythmias if the pacemaker fires during the T wave of the preceding beat.

PACEMAKER SYSTEM

The pacemaker system consists of a *pulse generator,* which houses the battery and controls various pacemaker functions, and an *electrode,* which

Understanding pacemakers

Temporary and permanent pacemakers are shown below. Although different models may vary slightly in appearance, they usually have the same features.

TEMPORARY PACEMAKER

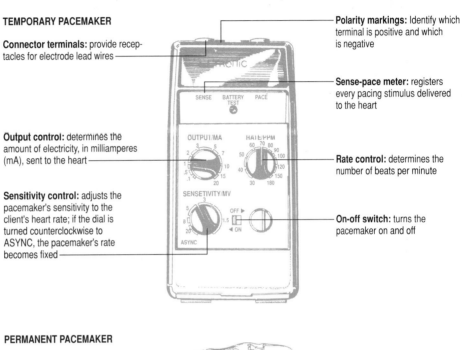

Connector terminals: provide receptacles for electrode lead wires

Output control: determines the amount of electricity, in milliamperes (mA), sent to the heart

Sensitivity control: adjusts the pacemaker's sensitivity to the client's heart rate; if the dial is turned counterclockwise to ASYNC, the pacemaker's rate becomes fixed

Polarity markings: Identify which terminal is positive and which is negative

Sense-pace meter: registers every pacing stimulus delivered to the heart

Rate control: determines the number of beats per minute

On-off switch: turns the pacemaker on and off

PERMANENT PACEMAKER

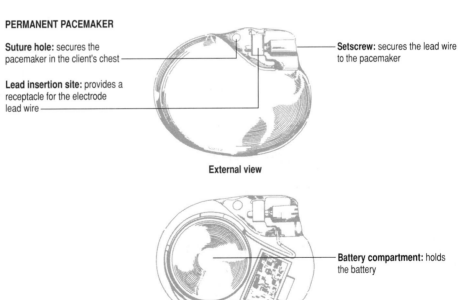

Suture hole: secures the pacemaker in the client's chest

Lead insertion site: provides a receptacle for the electrode lead wire

Setscrew: secures the lead wire to the pacemaker

External view

Battery compartment: holds the battery

Internal view

conducts the electrical impulse from the pulse generator to the client's heart. See *Understanding pacemakers,* page 179, for a discussion of permanent and temporary pulse generators. To learn the classification code for pacemaker systems, see *Pacemaker classification code,* page 182.

Types of electrodes   A bipolar electrode catheter has two pacemaker electrodes that come in contact with the endocardium. The bipolar catheter shown below is situated in the right ventricle.

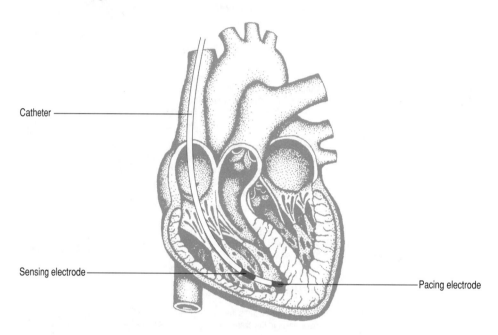

Catheter

Sensing electrode

Pacing electrode

The catheter's outside end is attached to the pulse generator. Inside the heart, the distal, or pacing, electrode at the catheter tip stimulates, or paces, the heart. The proximal, or sensing, electrode located about an inch farther up senses the heart's intrinsic rhythm. A demand pacemaker does not fire when the proximal electrode senses that the intrinsic heart rate is

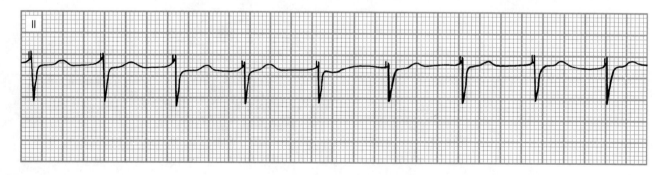

greater than the pacemaker's setting. Because of the short distance between the two electrodes, the pacing spike produced by a bipolar electrode catheter is small, as shown in the strip on the opposite page.

A unipolar electrode catheter has only one pacemaker electrode at its tip — the distal, or pacing, electrode. The proximal electrode is located in the pulse generator. Because the electrodes are so far apart, the pacing spike produced by a unipolar electrode catheter is large, as shown below.

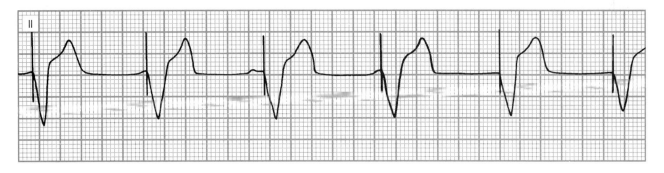

Electrical output The electrical output produced by a pulse generator to stimulate the heart is measured in milliamperes (mA). To select the appropriate output dial setting, the clinician must determine the pacing threshold. The pacing threshold is measured after the electrode catheter is correctly positioned in the heart and a pacing spike has produced an ECG complex and a heart beat. The output setting is then slowly decreased until the pacemaker no longer produces capture (an ECG complex and a heart beat). This setting is the pacing threshold, and an ECG reading at this output setting should be taken. The lower the reading, the more direct the contact between the catheter and the endocardium. The output is usually set at one and a half to three times the pacing threshold. High pacing thresholds can occur if the catheter is in poor contact with the endocardium, if scar tissue forms at the catheter site, or if the client has hypokalemia or suffers a myocardial infarction.

Hysteresis Hysteresis (a delay in the effect produced when forces acting on a body are changed) is a feature of newer pulse generators. Its purpose is to avoid competition between the client's intrinsic heart rate and the pacemaker's artificial heart rate. In hysteresis, the escape interval (time between the last beat of the intrinsic rhythm and the first paced beat) is longer than the paced interval (time between succeeding paced beats). Hysteresis is illustrated below.

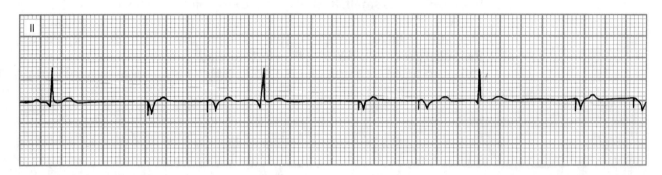

Response modes A pulse generator responds through inhibition or triggering. In the inhibition mode, the pacemaker turns off when the intrinsic rhythm rises above the paced interval. In the triggering mode, the pacemaker turns on in response to an intrinsic event. For example, in an atrial-ventricular pacemaker, the ventricular pacemaker may be triggered in response to a naturally occurring P wave that is not followed by a naturally occurring QRS complex.

I.C.H.D. CLASSIFICATION CODE

The Intersociety Commission on Heart Disease (ICHD) has developed a classification code for pacemaker systems. A three-letter code is usually used. The first letter corresponds to the chamber that is paced, the second letter to the chamber sensed, and the third letter to the response mode. For example, a VOO pacemaker paces the ventricle at a fixed rate. Commonly used pacemakers include VVI and DDD pacemakers.

Pacemaker classification code

Chamber paced	Chamber sensed	Response mode
A = Atrium	A = Atrium	I = Inhibited
V = Ventricle	V = Ventricle	T = Triggered
D = Dual (both atrium and ventricle)	D = Dual (both atrium and ventricle)	D = Dual (both triggered and inhibited)
	O = None (essentially a fixed-rate pacemaker)	O = None (seen in fixed-rate pacemakers)

VVI pacemaker   The VVI, the most commonly used pacemaker, has a bipolar electrode catheter positioned in the right ventricle. This demand pacemaker detects ventricular activity only, pacing the ventricle when intrinsic ventricular activity is not sensed. It is inhibited when intrinsic ventricular activity exceeds the rate of the paced interval. Because the impulse originates in the right ventricle, the pacemaker spike produces a wide and bizarre QRS complex similar to that seen in ventricular ectopic beats. The primary disadvantage of a VVI pacemaker is the loss of atrial activity and atrial kick, which can add 15% or more to the cardiac output. This lack of atrial kick, usually more of a problem in clients with heart failure or cardiomyopathy who already have a limited cardiac reserve, can result in pacemaker syndrome (see page 189).

The figure below shows an example of an ECG strip from a VVI pacemaker.

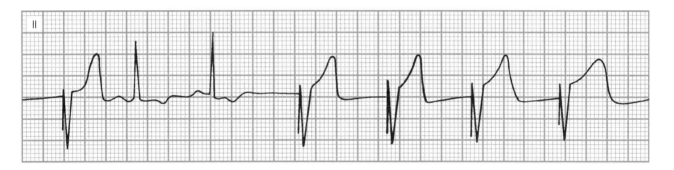

Use the following questions to evaluate the pacing of a VVI pacemaker:
- What is the rate of the paced rhythm?
- What is the rate of the intrinsic rhythm, if present?
- Is sensing appropriate?
- Is capture present at all times?

DDD pacemaker   The DDD pacemaker, also known as an atrial-ventricular sequential or dual-chamber pacemaker, sequentially paces the atrium and the ventricle on demand. An electrode catheter is situated in both the right atrium and the right ventricle, and sensing and pacing occur in both chambers (see *Dual-chamber pacing: Four variations,* page 184).

Dual-chamber pacing: Four variations

A dual-chamber pacemaker prevents the client's heart rate from dropping below the device's programmed level and ensures that ventricular contraction occurs shortly after atrial contraction. This pacemaker has been programmed at 80 beats/minute. The client's ECG strip may show any or all of the normal patterns below.

In this strip, the client's heart rate initially exceeds 80 beats/minute with no help, and the ventricles depolarize un-aided. Sensing no need for pacing of atria or ventricles, the pacemaker is inhibited from pacing.

Although the atrial rate is still faster than 80 beats/minute in this strip, the ventricles fail to depolarize by the end of the preprogrammed AV delay, so the pacemaker stimulates the ventricles. The shape of the QRS complex immediately changes when ventricular pacing begins.

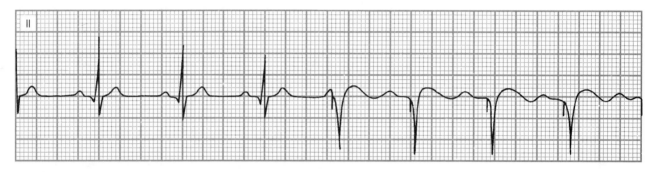

In this strip, atrial spikes from the pacemaker show that the atrial rate has slowed to 80 beats/minute, the pacemaker's programmed lower limit. Because the ventricles depolarize before completion of the AV delay, they need no stimulation.

When the client's intrinsic atrial rate remains too slow and the ventricles fail to depolarize before the preprogrammed AV delay deadline, as shown here, the pacemaker stimulates atria and ventricles, preventing a low heart rate and synchro-nizing atrial and ventricular contraction.

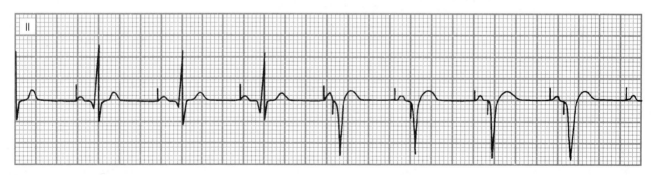

Adapted from Witherell, Charles, "Questions Nurses Ask About Pacemakers," *AJN*, December 1990. Used with permission.

If the escape interval elapses and no intrinsic atrial or ventricular activity is sensed, the atrial pulse generator paces the atrium. The ventricular pulse generator waits for intrinsic ventricular activity to follow an artificially controlled P-R interval called the AV delay, which is programmed into the pacemaker. If no intrinsic ventricular activity is sensed, the ventricular pulse generator paces the right ventricle. If intrinsic atrial activity occurs but intrinsic ventricular activity does not follow, the atrial pulse generator is inhibited by the atrial activity, while the ventricular pulse generator is triggered by the lack of intrinsic ventricular activity after the AV delay. The primary advantage of a DDD pacemaker is that normal atrial and ventricular filling occurs, thus maximizing cardiac output by retaining the atrial kick. The primary disadvantage is its complexity: the DDD is more difficult to insert than a VVI pacemaker.

Use the following questions to evaluate the pacing of a DDD pacemaker:
- What is the rate of the paced rhythm?
- What is the rate of the intrinsic rhythm?
- Is atrial sensing appropriate?
- Is atrial capture present?
- Is AV delay appropriate?
- Is ventricular sensing appropriate?
- Is ventricular capture present?

COMPLICATIONS OF PACING

Although pacemakers usually work effectively, they are not trouble-free. Potential complications include failure to sense, oversensing, failure to capture, failure to pace, microshock, myocardial perforation, pacemaker-mediated tachycardia, pacemaker syndrome, and arrhythmias.

Failure to sense   As shown in the rhythm strip below, a pacemaker may continue its attempts to pace the heart even though the client's intrinsic heart rate is

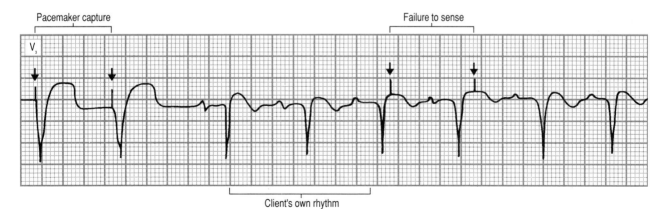

Pacemaker capture

Failure to sense

V₃

Client's own rhythm

above the escape interval. This complication produces pacing spikes that occur at inappropriate times during the client's intrinsic rhythm and that may compete with it.

The pacing spikes (identified by arrows) appear immediately after the QRS complexes. Such a pattern can occur if the catheter moves and the proximal electrode is no longer in a position to sense intrinsic activity. Failure to sense also can occur from battery failure, catheter fractures, or an incorrect setting (if the sensitivity control on a temporary pacemaker is switched to the fixed-rate, or asynchronous, mode).

Nursing implications
- Assess the pacemaker first — check the sensitivity control, and change the battery if needed.
- Ask the client to turn on the side; repositioning may move the catheter back into place.
- Prepare to administer an antiarrhythmic medication; ventricular arrhythmias can result if the pacing spikes fall on the T wave of the intrinsic beat.
- If the client's intrinsic heart rate is adequate and initial interventions have no effect, turn off the pacemaker until a physician can assess the problem.
- A chest X-ray may be required to determine whether the catheter has fractured, which would necessitate changing the catheter.

Oversensing
Oversensing occurs when the pacemaker, inhibited by a noncardiac stimulus, fires at a rate lower than the set rate. A common noncardiac stimulus is electromagnetic interference from cautery, diathermy, radiation therapy, or magnetic resonance imaging. Under such conditions, the pacemaker might mistake the electromagnetic interference for cardiac depolarization; this would inhibit the pacemaker from firing.

The figure below shows an example of oversensing, in which the pacemaker fires at a variable rate.

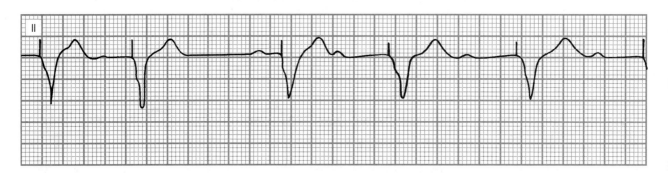

Nursing implications
- Check whether the pacemaker sensitivity control is set too high, and respond accordingly (a nurse is permitted to adjust this setting on a tem-

porary pacemaker, but a physician usually must reprogram a permanent pacemaker).
• If the problem does not resolve from adjusting the sensitivity setting, check for a source of electromagnetic interference.

Failure to capture Failure to capture may result from catheter movement, scarring at the contact site, battery failure, or catheter fracture. When capture fails to occur, the pacing spike appears at the appropriate time but a QRS complex does not follow.

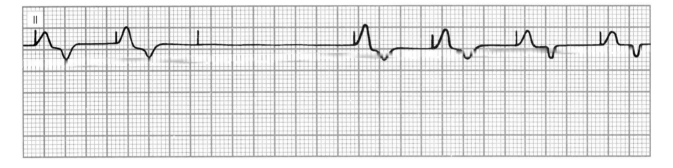

In this example, the third pacing spike is not followed by a QRS complex, indicating failure to capture.

Nursing implications • Increase the milliampere output slowly until capture occurs or the maximum setting is reached.
• If increasing the output is ineffective, replace the battery or reposition the client so that the catheter may move back to its correct position.

Failure to pace In failure to pace, the pacing spikes do not appear at the appropriate times. This complication can be caused by battery failure, catheter fracture, a disconnected catheter, or a power loss at the pulse generator. The figure below shows an example of failure to pace.

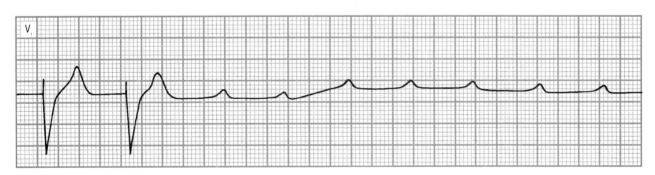

Nursing implications
- Ensure that the pulse generator is turned on.
- Replace the battery, if needed, and check all connections for tightness.

Microshock
An electrical current that comes in direct contact with the myocardium can produce microshock. A client with a temporary pacemaker is at risk for microshock because the pacemaker catheter provides direct access to the myocardium. Small amounts of current (1 to 5 mA) leaked directly into the heart can produce ventricular arrhythmias. Ungrounded or defective equipment may provide the electrical current that results in microshock.

Nursing implications
- Place the catheter terminals and the pulse generator in a rubber glove to insulate the catheter from microshock.
- Do not disconnect the catheter from the pulse generator; this would expose the catheter to electrical current from faulty equipment.
- If the catheter must be disconnected, wear rubber gloves and cover the catheter terminals with insulated tips.
- Prohibit the client from using ungrounded electrical equipment from home, such as an electric shaver, until it has been checked by the biomedical engineering department.
- Check all electrical equipment near the client for proper grounding, and have this equipment checked regularly by the biomedical engineering staff.
- Never touch electrical equipment and the client simultaneously; current could be transferred to the client.

Myocardial perforation
The pacemaker catheter can perforate the myocardium, resulting in minor complications (such as hiccups) or more severe conditions (such as myocardial hemorrhage and cardiac tamponade). Myocardial perforation is more likely to occur with a hardwire catheter, an older type of catheter that is sometimes used for clients in cardiac arrest when the lack of blood flow prevents insertion of a balloon-flotation catheter. A perforated myocardium usually results in loss of capture.

Nursing implications
- Suspect myocardial perforation if loss of capture is not resolved by initial interventions.
- Assess the client for signs and symptoms of cardiac tamponade, such as narrowing pulse pressure, hypotension, shortness of breath, enlarged cardiac silhouette on chest X-ray, and pulsus paradoxus.
- Reposition the catheter, if necessary.
- Prepare for emergency pericardiocentesis, if necessary.

Pacemaker-mediated tachycardia

Pacemaker-mediated tachycardia, also called endless-loop tachycardia, is a potential complication of a DDD pacemaker. A ventricular paced beat initiates retrograde atrial conduction, which triggers another ventricular paced beat. Tachycardia ensues, with a pacemaker spike preceding each QRS complex.

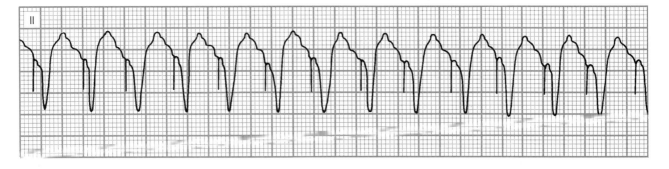

Nursing implications

• Notify a physician or a nurse who can reprogram the pacemaker so that the atrial sensing mechanism is interrupted, which will terminate the tachycardia.
• In an emergency, place a magnet over the pacemaker implantation site to convert the pacemaker to a fixed-rate mode, which also will terminate the tachycardia.
• Be prepared to administer an antiarrhythmic medication, and have emergency equipment available; ventricular tachycardia or ventricular fibrillation can occur before the pacemaker-mediated tachycardia resolves.

Pacemaker syndrome

Pacemaker syndrome can occur when a client with limited cardiac reserve receives a ventricular pacemaker. The loss of atrial kick decreases cardiac output, which can result in congestive heart failure.

Nursing implications

• Assess the client for weakness, fatigue, activity intolerance, weight gain, rales, and S_3 gallop.
• The preferred treatment for this syndrome is to replace the ventricular pacemaker with a DDD pacemaker.

Arrhythmias

Premature ventricular contractions (PVCs) are common in clients with a temporary pacemaker. They also occur during the immediate postoperative period in clients who have received a permanent pacemaker. Fibrous tissue begins to develop at the endocardial site within 24 hours after permanent pacemaker implantation, and irritation from the catheter disappears, which decreases the risk of PVCs. Lethal ventricular arrhythmias can be initiated by the pacemaker's failure to sense.

Nursing implications
- • PVCs are not usually treated. If PVCs become frequent and episodes of ventricular tachycardia develop, administer an antiarrhythmic drug, as prescribed.
- • Prepare to reposition the catheter of a temporary pacemaker.

FUSION BEATS

Although they may appear to be a complication of pacemaker therapy, fusion beats occur benignly when the pacemaker and the client's intrinsic conduction system activate the heart simultaneously. Fusion beats are preceded by a pacing spike, but the QRS complex that follows the spike usually looks like the client's intrinsic rhythm. The 5th and 6th QRS complexes in the figure below are examples of fusion beats.

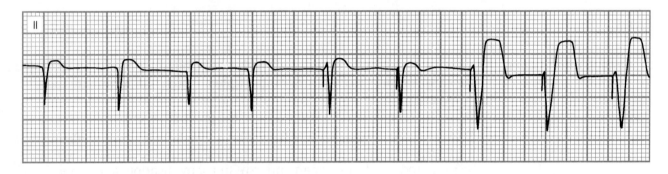

PRACTICE EXAMPLE

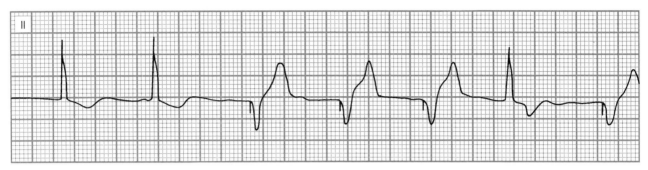

ECG characteristics   *Rate of paced rhythm:*

Rate of intrinsic rhythm:

Pacing in atrium, ventricle, or both?

Is sensing appropriate?

Is capture present?

Fusion beats?

Arrhythmias?

Interpretation   _____

_____

Treatment   _____

_____

_____

_____

_____

_____

ANSWER TO PRACTICE EXAMPLE

PACED RHYTHMS

ECG characteristics

Rate of paced rhythm: 72 beats/minute
Rate of intrinsic rhythm: 72 beats/minute
Pacing in atrium, ventricle, or both? Ventricle
Is sensing appropriate? Yes
Is capture present? Yes
Fusion beats? No
Arrhythmias? No

Interpretation   Demand ventricular pacing with 100% capture

Treatment   Continue to observe for proper sensing and capture.

SELF – TESTS

You can verify your understanding of the material presented in this chapter by completing the following self-tests. Like the practice example, the self-tests will assess your knowledge of ECG characteristics, rhythm interpretation, and treatments. Complete all three self-tests in this chapter before comparing your responses with the correct answers in Appendix A, pages 212 and 213.

SELF – TEST 1

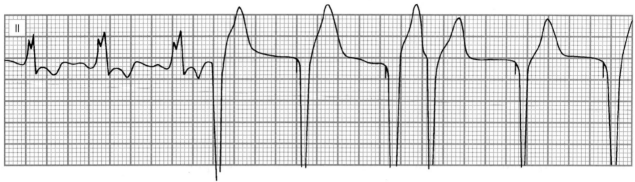

ECG characteristics   *Rate of paced rhythm:*

_____

Rate of intrinsic rhythm:

_____

Pacing in atrium, ventricle, or both?

_____

Is sensing appropriate?

_____

Is capture present?

_____

Fusion beats?

_____

Arrhythmias?

_____

Interpretation _____

_____

Treatment _____

_____

_____

_____

_____

SELF – TEST 2

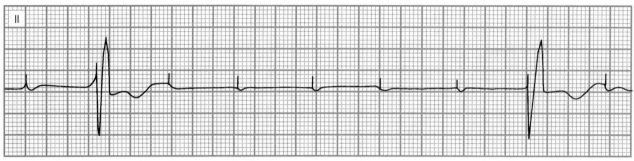

ECG characteristics

Rate of paced rhythm:

_____

Rate of intrinsic rhythm:

_____

Pacing in atrium, ventricle, or both?

_____

Is sensing appropriate?

_____

Is capture present?

_____

Fusion beats?

_____

Arrhythmias?

_____

Interpretation

Treatment

SELF – TEST 3

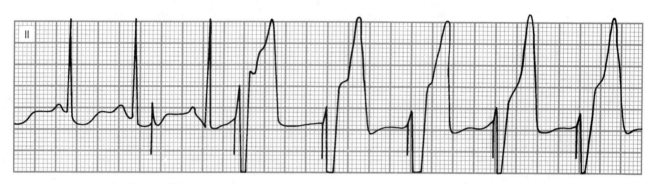

ECG characteristics

Rate of paced rhythm:

_____

Rate of intrinsic rhythm:

_____

Pacing in atrium, ventricle, or both?

_____

Is sensing appropriate?

_____

Is capture present?

_____

Fusion beats?

_____

Arrhythmias?

_____

Interpretation _____

_____

Treatment _____

_____

_____

_____

_____

_____

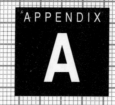

APPENDIX

A

Answers to Self–Tests

CHAPTER 3: SINUS ARRHYTHMIAS 1

ECG characteristics

P wave *Configuration:* All normal and alike, except for an absent P wave and QRS complex between the 6th and 7th impulses
Rate: About 80 beats/minute
Rhythm: Regular, except for the pause

P-R interval 0.16 second

QRS complex *Configuration:* All normal and alike
Rate: About 80 beats/minute
Rhythm: Regular, except for the pause, which is twice the normal R-R interval
Duration: 0.08 second

Interpretation Sinus exit block (because the pause is a multiple of the R-R interval)

Treatment If pauses become longer and cause hypotension, dizziness, or syncope, administer atropine 0.5 mg I.V. every 5 minutes to a maximum dosage of 2 mg. If symptoms persist, administer isoproterenol 2 to 10 mcg/minute until a pacemaker is inserted.

Nursing implications
- Continue to observe the client for further pauses.
- Monitor the client's digoxin level.
- Assess the client for signs and symptoms of decreased cardiac output, such as hypotension and decreased level of consciousness.

CHAPTER 3: SINUS ARRHYTHMIAS 2

ECG characteristics

P wave *Configuration:* All upright, normal, and alike
Rate: About 30 beats/minute
Rhythm: Irregular

P-R interval 0.18 second

QRS complex *Configuration:* All normal and alike
Rate: About 30 beats/minute
Rhythm: Irregular; 0.18 second between R-R intervals
Duration: 0.08 second

Interpretation Sinus bradycardia with an irregular rhythm

Treatment If the client develops syncope or hypotension, administer atropine 0.5 mg I.V. every 5 minutes to a maximum dosage of 2 mg. If symptoms persist, administer isoproterenol 2 to 10 mcg/minute until a pacemaker is inserted.

Nursing implications
- Monitor the client's digoxin level.
- Assess the client for signs and symptoms of decreased cardiac output, such as hypotension and decreased level of consciousness.

CHAPTER 3: SINUS ARRHYTHMIAS 3

ECG characteristics

P wave *Configuration:* All normal, upright, and alike
Rate: 130 beats/minute
Rhythm: Regular

P-R interval 0.16 second

QRS complex *Configuration:* All normal and alike
Rate: 130 beats/minute
Rhythm: Regular
Duration: 0.08 second

Interpretation Sinus tachycardia

Treatment Therapy focuses on identifying and treating the underlying cause, such as fever, pain, or hypoxia.

Nursing implications
- Determine what is causing the sinus tachycardia.
- Use independent nursing actions, such as rest and relaxation techniques, to resolve the arrhythmia.

CHAPTER 4: ATRIAL ARRHYTHMIAS 1

ECG characteristics

P wave *Configuration:* All P waves are normal and alike, except for one premature P wave (after the 7th QRS complex) that is buried in a T wave
Rate: About 90 beats/minute
Rhythm: Regular except for the 7th P wave, which is premature

P-R interval 0.18 second

QRS complex *Configuration:* All QRS complexes are normal and alike, except for the dropped QRS complex after the 7th P wave

Rate: About 80 beats/minute
Rhythm: Regular except for the dropped QRS complex
Duration: 0.08 second

Interpretation Normal sinus rhythm with one nonconducted premature atrial contraction (PAC)

Treatment No treatment is needed. However, if the PACs occur more frequently and are not caused by digoxin toxicity, then digoxin may be administered, alone or in combination with quinidine.

Nursing implications
- Explain to the client how caffeine, alcohol, and stress can contribute to PACs. Recommend limited or restricted caffeine and alcohol intake, and teach new relaxation techniques.
- Monitor the client's serum potassium and digoxin levels; withhold digoxin if serum levels are elevated.
- Observe the ECG monitor for increased frequency of PACs, which may signal the onset of more severe atrial arrhythmias.

CHAPTER 4: ATRIAL ARRHYTHMIAS 2

ECG characteristics
P wave *Configuration:* All normal and alike; two P waves are seen for each QRS complex
Rate: 180 beats/minute
Rhythm: Regular

P-R interval 0.18 second

QRS complex *Configuration:* All normal and alike
Rate: 90 beats/minute
Rhythm: Regular
Duration: 0.10 second

Interpretation Atrial tachycardia with 2:1 conduction block

Treatment The ventricular rate is normal; no immediate treatment is needed.

Nursing implications Monitor the client's serum digoxin level; withhold digoxin if indicated.

CHAPTER 4: ATRIAL ARRHYTHMIAS 3

ECG characteristics

P wave   *Configuration:* Wavy baseline
Rate: Not measurable
Rhythm: Irregular

P-R interval   Not measurable

QRS complex   *Configuration:* Normal and alike
Rate: About 90 beats/minute
Rhythm: Irregular
Duration: 0.08 second

Interpretation   Atrial fibrillation

Treatment   Pharmacologic therapy may include:
- digoxin 0.25 mg by mouth daily
- quinidine sulfate 200 mg by mouth every 3 to 4 hours or quinidine gluconate 324 mg by mouth every 6 to 8 hours
- procainamide 250 to 500 mg by mouth every 3 hours; for the slow-release form (Procan SR), 500 mg to 1 g every 6 hours
- propranolol 10 to 40 mg by mouth four times daily
- verapamil 80 mg by mouth three times daily.

Nursing implications
- Assess the client for signs of congestive heart failure, such as rales, dyspnea, and an S_3 gallop.
- Monitor the client's serum potassium and digoxin levels; withhold digoxin if serum levels are elevated.

CHAPTER 4: ATRIAL ARRHYTHMIAS 4

ECG characteristics

P wave   *Configuration:* P waves look dissimilar; one P wave appears for each QRS complex
Rate: About 70 beats/minute
Rhythm: Irregular

P-R interval   Varies from 0.14 to 0.20 second

QRS complex   *Configuration:* Normal and alike
Rate: About 70 beats/minute
Rhythm: Irregular
Duration: 0.06 second

Interpretation	Wandering atrial pacemaker
Treatment	No treatment is needed unless the client develops digoxin toxicity.
Nursing implications	• Monitor the client's serum digoxin level; withhold digoxin if the serum level is elevated. • Assess the client for bradycardia and hypotension.

CHAPTER 5: JUNCTIONAL ARRHYTHMIAS 1

ECG characteristics	
P wave	*Configuration:* Normal and alike, with one P wave preceding each QRS complex *Rate:* 80 beats/minute *Rhythm:* Regular
P-R interval	0.10 second
QRS complex	*Configuration:* All normal and alike *Rate:* 80 beats/minute *Rhythm:* Regular *Duration:* 0.08 second
Interpretation	Accelerated junctional rhythm
Treatment	No treatment is needed. Administer atropine if the client's heart rate decreases and hypotension or syncope develops.
Nursing implications	• Monitor the client's serum digoxin level; withhold digoxin, if indicated. • Consult the physician about discontinuing any antiarrhythmic agents.

CHAPTER 5: JUNCTIONAL ARRHYTHMIAS 2

ECG characteristics	
P wave	*Configuration:* All normal and alike except for the 2nd P wave from the end, which is inverted *Rate:* 75 beats/minute *Rhythm:* Regular except for one premature beat
P-R interval	0.20 second
QRS complex	*Configuration:* All normal and alike *Rate:* 75 beats/minute

Rhythm: Regular except for one premature beat
Duration: 0.08 second

Interpretation   Normal sinus rhythm with one premature junctional contraction (PJC)

Treatment   No treatment is needed.

Nursing implications
- Monitor the client's serum digoxin level. PJCs can result from digoxin toxicity.
- Explain how caffeine can contribute to PJCs, and urge the client to eliminate it from the diet or restrict its use.

CHAPTER 5: JUNCTIONAL ARRHYTHMIAS 3

ECG characteristics
P wave   *Configuration:* No P waves are visible
Rate: Not measurable
Rhythm: Not measurable

P-R interval   Not measurable

QRS complex   *Configuration:* All normal and alike
Rate: 52 beats/minute
Rhythm: Regular
Duration: 0.08 second

Interpretation   Junctional rhythm

Treatment   If the client develops syncope or hypotension, administer atropine 0.5 mg I.V. every 5 minutes up to the maximum dosage of 2 mg. If necessary, a temporary pacemaker may be inserted.

Nursing implications   Monitor the client's serum digoxin level; withhold digoxin, if indicated.

CHAPTER 6: VENTRICULAR ARRHYTHMIAS 1

ECG characteristics
P wave   *Configuration:* None
Rate: None
Rhythm: None

P-R interval   None

QRS complex   *Configuration:* Wide and bizarre

Rate: 240 beats/minute
Rhythm: Regular
Duration: 0.24 second

Interpretation   Ventricular tachycardia

Treatment   If the episode is witnessed, administer a precordial thump. If the client is conscious and hemodynamically stable:
- administer lidocaine 1 mg/kg I.V. followed by 0.5 mg/kg every 5 minutes to a maximum dosage of 3 mg; a continuous infusion of 2 to 4 mg/minute follows
- administer procainamide 50 mg/minute I.V. until a maximum dosage of 1 g is reached, the arrhythmia subsides, or the QRS complex widens by at least 50%; a continuous infusion of 1 to 4 mg/minute follows (procainamide is administered if lidocaine proves ineffective)
- administer bretylium 5 to 10 mg/kg followed by a continuous infusion of 1 to 2 mg/minute (bretylium is administered if lidocaine and procainamide prove ineffective)
- administer synchronized cardioversion at 50 to 100 watts/second and repeat, if necessary, at 200, 200 to 300, and 360 watts/second. Sedate a conscious client before cardioversion.

   If the client is unconscious or hemodynamically unstable:
- administer synchronized or unsynchronized cardioversion first, then antiarrhythmic agents.

   If the client has no pulse:
- defibrillate at 200 watts/second and increase to 300 then 360 watts/second if the initial attempt is unsuccessful
- perform cardiopulmonary resuscitation between defibrillation attempts
- administer antiarrhythmic drugs and epinephrine 0.5 to 1 mg every 5 minutes followed by defibrillation at the maximum 360 watts/second until the arrhythmia is terminated.

Nursing implications   Assess the client quickly to determine the appropriate treatment.

CHAPTER 6: VENTRICULAR ARRHYTHMIAS 2

ECG characteristics
   P wave   *Configuration:* Normal and alike when visible; one P wave before each normal QRS complex, no P waves before abnormal QRS complexes
Rate: 47 beats/minute
Rhythm: Regular

P-R interval   0.16 second

QRS complex	*Configuration:* Sinus beats are normal and alike; every other beat is wide and bizarre

QRS complex   *Configuration:* Sinus beats are normal and alike; every other beat is wide and bizarre
Rate: Approximately 90 beats/minute
Rhythm: Regularly irregular; every other beat is premature
Duration: 0.08 second for normal beats; 0.12 second for abnormal beats

Interpretation   Sinus rhythm with ventricular bigeminy

Treatment   Pharmacologic therapy may include:
- lidocaine 1 mg/kg I.V. followed by 0.5 mg/kg every 5 minutes to a maximum dosage of 3 mg; a continuous infusion of 2 to 4 mg/minute follows
- procainamide 50 mg/minute I.V. until a maximum dosage of 1 g is reached, the arrhythmia subsides, or the QRS complex widens by at least 50%; a continuous infusion of 1 to 4 mg/minute follows (procainamide is administered if lidocaine proves ineffective)
- bretylium 5 to 10 mg/kg followed by a continuous infusion of 1 to 2 mg/minute (bretylium is administered if lidocaine and procainamide prove ineffective).

Nursing implications
- Know the institution's policy on standing orders for lidocaine administration.
- Monitor the client's arterial blood gas values and serum digoxin and potassium levels.
- Administer supplemental oxygen, as prescribed.
- Place the client on a cardiac monitor, and use an infusion pump for medication administration.

CHAPTER 6: VENTRICULAR ARRHYTHMIAS 3

ECG characteristics
P wave   *Configuration:* None
Rate: None
Rhythm: None

P-R interval   None

QRS complex   *Configuration:* Wavy baseline
Rate: Rapid; cannot be determined precisely
Rhythm: Completely irregular
Duration: None

Interpretation   Ventricular fibrillation

Treatment Administer a precordial thump if you witness the episode. Defibrillate the client at 200 watts/second and increase to 300 then 360 watts/second if the initial attempt is unsuccessful. Perform cardiopulmonary resuscitation between defibrillation attempts. Pharmacologic therapy may include:
- epinephrine 0.5 to 1 mg I.V. every 5 minutes followed by defibrillation at 360 watts/second
- lidocaine 1 mg/kg I.V. followed by 0.5 mg/kg every 5 minutes to a maximum dosage of 3 mg; a continuous infusion of 2 to 4 mg/minute follows
- bretylium 5 to 10 mg/kg followed by a continuous infusion of 1 to 2 mg/minute (bretylium is administered if lidocaine proves ineffective).

Nursing implications
- Prompt recognition of ventricular fibrillation and treatment with defibrillation are crucial to successful therapy.
- Use a manual resuscitation bag with 100% oxygen to support the client's airway during defibrillation.

CHAPTER 6: VENTRICULAR ARRHYTHMIAS 4

ECG characteristics
P wave *Configuration:* Visible after the QRS complexes because of retrograde conduction
Rate: About 40 beats/minute
Rhythm: Irregular

P-R interval Not measurable

QRS complex *Configuration:* Wide and bizarre
Rate: About 40 beats/minute
Rhythm: Irregular
Duration: 0.12 second

Interpretation Idioventricular rhythm

Treatment Administer atropine 0.5 mg I.V. every 5 minutes to a maximum dosage of 2 mg. A temporary pacemaker may be necessary. Administer isoproterenol 2 to 10 mcg/minute after the maximum atropine dosage has been given and until a pacemaker is inserted.

Nursing implications
- Know the institution's policy on standing orders for atropine administration.
- Monitor the client's serum digoxin and potassium levels.
- Discontinue any lidocaine infusion.

CHAPTER 7: ATRIOVENTRICULAR BLOCKS 1

ECG characteristics

P wave   *Configuration:* All normal and alike; every other P wave is not associated with a QRS complex
Rate: 66 beats/minute
Rhythm: Regular

P-R interval   0.20 second

QRS complex   *Configuration:* All normal and alike
Rate: 30 beats/minute
Rhythm: Regular
Duration: 0.10 second

Interpretation   Second-degree AV block, Mobitz type II, with a 2:1 conduction ratio

Treatment   Administer atropine 0.5 mg I.V. every 5 minutes to a maximum dosage of 2 mg. A temporary pacemaker may be necessary. Administer isoproterenol 2 to 10 mcg/minute after the maximum atropine dosage has been given and until a pacemaker is inserted.

Nursing implications   • Prepare for pacemaker insertion, if indicated.
• Place the client in a supine position to reverse hypotension.
• Monitor the client's serum digoxin level, if indicated.
• Administer supplemental oxygen, as needed.

CHAPTER 7: ATRIOVENTRICULAR BLOCKS 2

ECG characteristics

P wave   *Configuration:* All normal and alike; one P wave appears for each QRS complex
Rate: 75 beats/minute
Rhythm: Regular

P-R interval   0.28 second

QRS complex   *Configuration:* All normal and alike
Rate: 75 beats/minute
Rhythm: Regular
Duration: 0.08 second

Interpretation   First-degree AV block

Treatment   No treatment is needed because the ventricular rate is within normal limits.

Nursing implications
- Monitor the client's serum digoxin level, if indicated.
- Assess the client for more severe degrees of AV block.

CHAPTER 7: ATRIOVENTRICULAR BLOCKS 3

ECG characteristics

P wave   *Configuration:* All normal and alike; the ratio of P waves to QRS complexes is 3:2
Rate: 69 beats/minute
Rhythm: Regular

P-R interval   Varies from 0.26 second to 0.38 second, lengthening progressively

QRS complex   *Configuration:* All normal and alike
Rate: About 40 beats/minute
Rhythm: Irregular
Duration: 0.08 second

Interpretation   Second-degree AV block, Mobitz type I

Treatment   Administer atropine 0.5 mg I.V. every 5 minutes to a maximum dosage of 2 mg. A temporary pacemaker may be necessary. Administer isoproterenol 2 to 10 mcg/minute after the maximum atropine dosage has been given and until a pacemaker is inserted.

Nursing implications
- Prepare for pacemaker insertion, if indicated.
- Place the client in a supine position to reverse hypotension.
- Monitor the client's serum digoxin level, if indicated.
- Administer supplemental oxygen, as needed.

CHAPTER 7: ATRIOVENTRICULAR BLOCKS 4

ECG characteristics

P wave   *Configuration:* Normal and alike; P waves march through the QRS complexes
Rate: 100 beats/minute
Rhythm: Regular

P-R interval   No identifiable pattern emerges

QRS complex	*Configuration:* Wide and alike
	Rate: About 30 beats/minute
	Rhythm: Regular
	Duration: 0.12 second

Interpretation   Third-degree AV block

Treatment   Administer atropine 0.5 mg I.V. every 5 minutes up to 2 mg. A temporary pacemaker may be necessary. Administer isoproterenol 2 to 10 mcg/minute after the maximum atropine dosage has been given and until a pacemaker is inserted.

Nursing implications
- Immediately prepare for pacemaker insertion.
- Place the client in a supine position to reverse hypotension.
- Monitor the client's serum digoxin level, if indicated.
- Administer supplemental oxygen, as needed.

CHAPTER 8: PACED RHYTHMS 1

ECG characteristics   *Rate of paced rhythm:* 72 beats/minute
Rate of intrinsic rhythm: 85 beats/minute
Pacing in atrium, ventricle, or both? Ventricle
Is sensing appropriate? Yes
Is capture present? Yes
Fusion beats? No
Arrhythmias? One premature ventricular contraction (PVC) after the 3rd paced beat

Interpretation   Demand ventricular pacing with 100% capture; one PVC seen

Treatment   Continue to observe for proper sensing and capture. Administer an antiarrhythmic medication if PVCs become frequent.

CHAPTER 8: PACED RHYTHMS 2

ECG characteristics   *Rate of paced rhythm:* 90 beats/minute
Rate of intrinsic rhythm: None measurable
Pacing in atrium, ventricle, or both? Ventricle
Is sensing appropriate? Yes
Is capture present? No, except for two beats
Fusion beats? No
Arrhythmias? No

Interpretation   Ventricular pacing without capture

Treatment   Increase the milliampere output. Turn the client on the side to reposition the catheter. Replace the pacemaker battery.

CHAPTER 8: PACED RHYTHMS 3

ECG characteristics   *Rate of paced rhythm:* 75 beats/minute
Rate of intrinsic rhythm: About 95 beats/minute
Pacing in atrium, ventricle, or both? Ventricle
Is sensing appropriate? No; second and third intrinsic beats are not sensed
Is capture present? Yes, except for one failure after the second intrinsic beat, because the myocardium is absolutely refractory
Fusion beats? No
Arrhythmias? No

Interpretation   Demand ventricular pacing with failure to sense

Treatment   Check the sensitivity control on the pulse generator and adjust if necessary. Replace the pacemaker battery. Turn the client on the side to reposition the catheter.

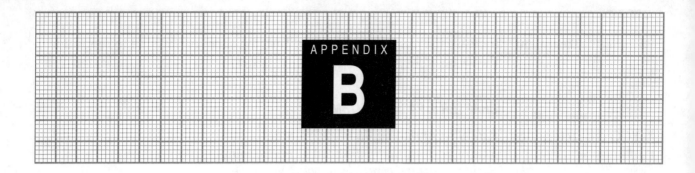

APPENDIX

B

Post–Tests and Answers

POST – TEST 1

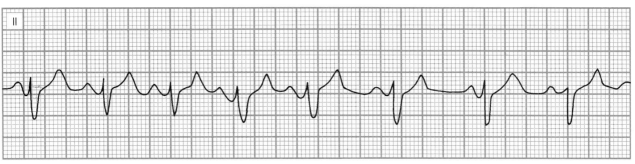

ECG characteristics

P wave   *Configuration:*

Rate:

Rhythm:

P-R interval

QRS complex   *Configuration:*

Rate:

Rhythm:

Duration:

Interpretation _____

_____

Treatment _____

_____

_____

_____

_____

_____

Nursing implications _____

_____

_____

_____

_____

_____

_____

POST – TEST 2

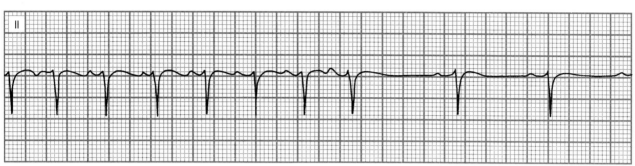

ECG characteristics

P wave *Configuration:* _____

_____

Rate: _____

_____

Rhythm: _____

_____

P-R interval _____

_____

QRS complex *Configuration:* _____

_____

Rate: _____

_____

Rhythm: _____

_____

Duration: _____

_____

Interpretation _____

_____

Treatment _____

_____

_____

_____

_____

_____

Nursing implications _____

_____

_____

_____

_____

_____

POST – TEST 3

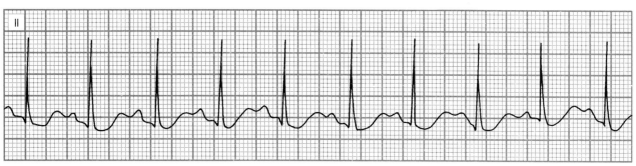

ECG characteristics

P wave *Configuration:*
_____

_____

Rate:
_____

_____

Rhythm:
_____

_____

P-R interval
_____

_____

QRS complex *Configuration:*
_____

_____

Rate:
_____

_____

Rhythm:
_____

_____

Duration:
_____

_____

Interpretation _____

_____

Treatment _____

_____

_____

_____

_____

_____

Nursing implications _____

_____

_____

_____

_____

_____

POST – TEST 4

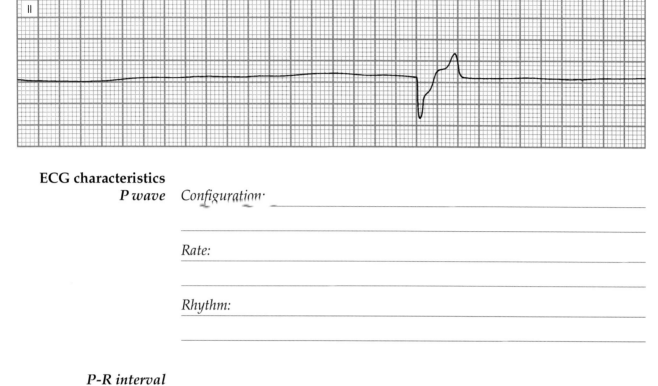

ECG characteristics

P wave   *Configuration:* _____

_____

Rate: _____

_____

Rhythm: _____

_____

P-R interval   _____

_____

QRS complex   *Configuration:* _____

_____

Rate: _____

_____

Rhythm: _____

_____

Duration: _____

_____

Interpretation _____

_____

Treatment _____

_____

_____

_____

_____

_____

Nursing implications _____

_____

_____

_____

_____

_____

_____

POST – TEST 5

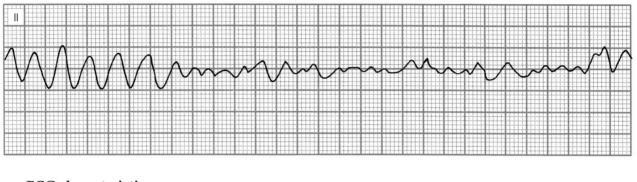

ECG characteristics

P wave   *Configuration:*

_____

_____

Rate:

_____

_____

Rhythm:

_____

_____

P-R interval

_____

_____

QRS complex   *Configuration:*

_____

_____

Rate:

_____

_____

Rhythm:

_____

_____

Duration:

_____

_____

Interpretation _____

_____

Treatment _____

_____

_____

_____

_____

_____

Nursing implications _____

_____

_____

_____

_____

_____

POST – TEST 6

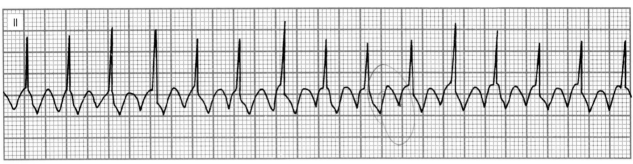

ECG characteristics

P wave Configuration: _____

_____

Rate: _____

_____

Rhythm: _____

_____

P-R interval _____

_____

QRS complex Configuration: _____

_____

Rate: _____

_____

Rhythm: _____

_____

Duration: _____

_____

Interpretation _____
_____

Treatment _____
_____
_____
_____
_____
_____

Nursing implications _____
_____
_____
_____
_____
_____

POST – TEST 7

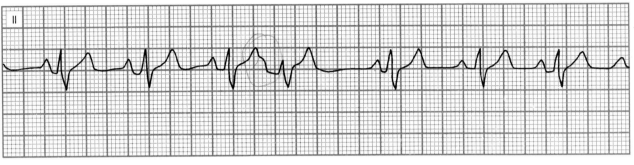

ECG characteristics

P wave   *Configuration.*

            Rate:

            Rhythm:

P-R interval

QRS complex   *Configuration:*

            Rate:

            Rhythm:

            Duration:

Interpretation   _____

_____

Treatment   _____

_____

_____

_____

_____

_____

Nursing implications   _____

_____

_____

_____

_____

_____

_____

POST – TEST 8

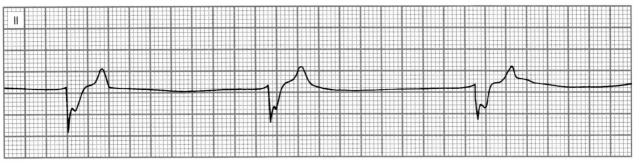

ECG characteristics

P wave   *Configuration:* _____

_____

Rate: _____

_____

Rhythm: _____

_____

P-R interval   _____

_____

QRS complex   *Configuration:* _____

_____

Rate: _____

_____

Rhythm: _____

_____

Duration: _____

_____

Interpretation   _____

_____

Treatment   _____

_____

_____

_____

_____

_____

Nursing implications   _____

_____

_____

_____

_____

_____

_____

POST – TEST 9

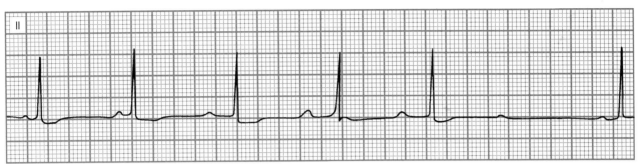

ECG characteristics

P wave   *Configuration:*

_____

Rate:

_____

Rhythm:

_____

P-R interval

_____

QRS complex   *Configuration:*

_____

Rate:

_____

Rhythm:

_____

Duration:

_____

Interpretation _____

_____

Treatment _____

_____

_____

_____

_____

_____

Nursing implications _____

_____

_____

_____

_____

_____

POST – TEST 10

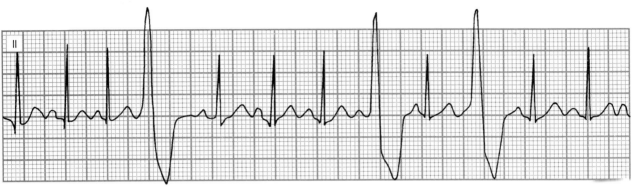

ECG characteristics

P wave *Configuration:*
_____

_____

Rate:
_____

_____

Rhythm:
_____

_____

P-R interval
_____

_____

QRS complex *Configuration:*
_____

_____

Rate:
_____

Rhythm:
_____

Duration:
_____

_____

Interpretation _____

_____

Treatment _____

_____

_____

_____

_____

_____

Nursing implications _____

_____

_____

_____

_____

_____

_____

POST – TEST 11

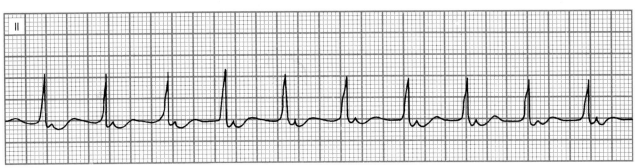

ECG characteristics

P wave   Configuration:

Rate:

Rhythm:

P-R interval

QRS complex   Configuration:

Rate:

Rhythm:

Duration:

Interpretation _____

_____

Treatment _____

_____

_____

_____

_____

_____

Nursing implications _____

_____

_____

_____

_____

_____

POST – TEST 12

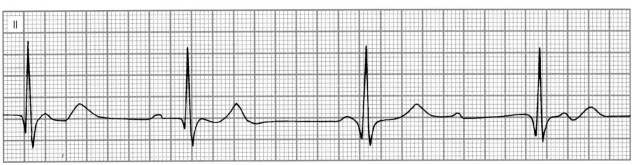

ECG characteristics

P wave   *Configuration:*

_____

Rate:

_____

Rhythm:

_____

P-R interval

_____

_____

QRS complex   *Configuration:*

_____

Rate:

_____

Rhythm:

_____

Duration:

_____

Interpretation _____

_____

Treatment _____

_____

_____

_____

_____

_____

Nursing implications _____

_____

_____

_____

_____

_____

POST – TEST 13

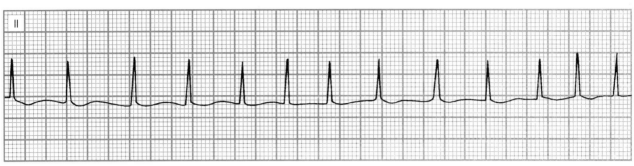

ECG characteristics

P wave Configuration: _____

Rate: _____

Rhythm: _____

P-R interval _____

QRS complex Configuration: _____

Rate: _____

Rhythm: _____

Duration: _____

Interpretation   _____

_____

Treatment   _____

_____

_____

_____

_____

_____

Nursing implications   _____

_____

_____

_____

_____

_____

POST – TEST 14

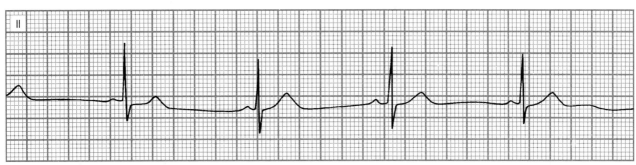

ECG characteristics

P wave   *Configuration:* _____

_____

Rate: _____

_____

Rhythm: _____

_____

P-R interval   _____

_____

QRS complex   *Configuration:* _____

_____

Rate: _____

_____

Rhythm: _____

_____

Duration: _____

_____

Interpretation
_____

_____

Treatment
_____

_____

_____

_____

_____

_____

Nursing implications
_____

_____

_____

_____

_____

_____

POST – TEST 15

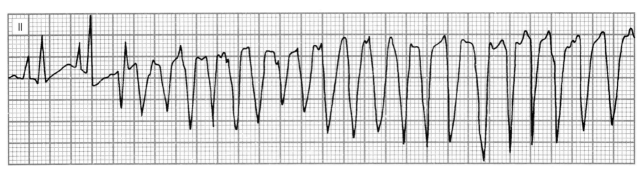

ECG characteristics

P wave   *Configuration:*
_____

_____

Rate:
_____

_____

Rhythm:
_____

_____

P-R interval
_____

_____

QRS complex   *Configuration:*
_____

_____

Rate:
_____

_____

Rhythm:
_____

_____

Duration:
_____

_____

Interpretation

_____

_____

Treatment

_____

_____

_____

_____

_____

_____

Nursing implications

_____

_____

_____

_____

_____

_____

POST – TEST 16

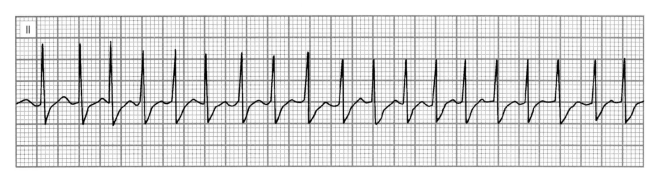

ECG characteristics

P wave   *Configuration:*

Rate:

Rhythm:

P-R interval

QRS complex   *Configuration:*

Rate:

Rhythm:

Duration:

Interpretation _____

_____

Treatment _____

_____

_____

_____

_____

_____

Nursing implications _____

_____

_____

_____

_____

_____

POST – TEST 17

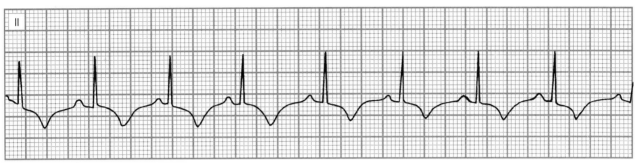

ECG characteristics

P wave *Configuration:*

_____

_____

Rate:

_____

_____

Rhythm:

_____

_____

P-R interval

_____

_____

QRS complex *Configuration:*

_____

_____

Rate:

_____

_____

Rhythm:

_____

_____

Duration:

_____

_____

Interpretation _____

_____

Treatment _____

_____

_____

_____

_____

_____

Nursing implications _____

_____

_____

_____

_____

_____

POST – TEST 18

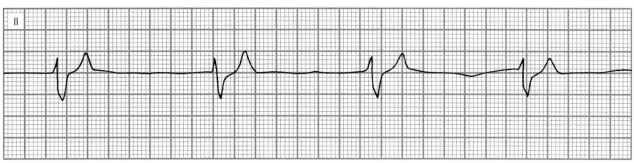

ECG characteristics

   P wave *Configuration:*

        Rate:

        Rhythm:

  P-R interval

 QRS complex *Configuration:*

        Rate:

        Rhythm:

        Duration:

Interpretation _____

_____

Treatment _____

_____

_____

_____

_____

_____

Nursing implications _____

_____

_____

_____

_____

_____

POST – TEST 19

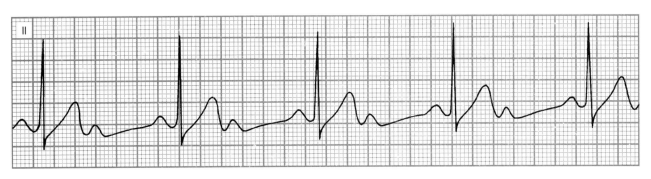

ECG characteristics

P wave   Configuration:

Rate:

Rhythm:

P-R interval

QRS complex   Configuration:

Rate:

Rhythm:

Duration:

Interpretation _____

_____

Treatment _____

_____

_____

_____

_____

_____

Nursing implications _____

_____

_____

_____

_____

_____

POST – TEST 20

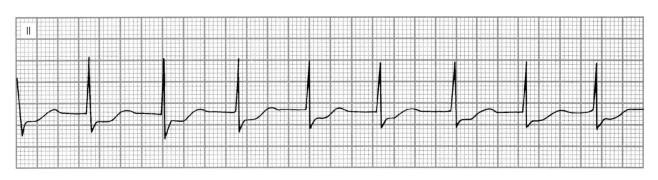

ECG characteristics

P wave   *Configuration:*

_____

Rate:

_____

Rhythm:

_____

P-R interval

_____

QRS complex   *Configuration:*

_____

Rate:

_____

Rhythm:

_____

Duration:

_____

Interpretation _____

_____

Treatment _____

_____

_____

_____

_____

_____

Nursing implications _____

_____

_____

_____

_____

_____

ANSWERS TO POST – TESTS

POST – TEST 1

ECG characteristics

P wave   *Configuration:* All upright, normal, and alike
Rate: Approximately 80 beats/minute
Rhythm: Irregular

P-R interval   0.20 second

QRS complex   *Configuration:* All alike but slightly wide
Rate: About 80 beats/minute
Rhythm: Irregular; the difference between the shortest (2nd-3rd complexes) and the longest (6th-7th complexes) R-R interval is 0.24 second
Duration: 0.12 second

Interpretation   Sinus arrhythmia with a ventricular conduction delay

Treatment   No treatment is needed.

Nursing implications   Continue to observe and monitor the client.

POST – TEST 2

ECG characteristics

P wave   *Configuration:* All normal and alike except for the P wave that precedes the termination of the tachycardia
Rate: Varies from 130 to 69 beats/minute
Rhythm: The tachycardia is regular and terminated by a premature beat; the sinus rhythm is regular

P-R interval   0.18 second

QRS complex   *Configuration:* All normal and alike
Rate: Varies from 130 to 69 beats/minute
Rhythm: Same as the atrial rhythm
Duration: 0.08 second

Interpretation   Paroxysmal atrial tachycardia terminated by a premature atrial contraction, then normal sinus rhythm

Treatment   If paroxysmal atrial tachycardia returns, prepare for carotid sinus massage, synchronized cardioversion at 50 to 100 watts/second, or overdrive pacing. Pharmacologic therapy may include:

- digoxin 0.25 to 0.50 mg I.V.
- propranolol 1 mg I.V. every 5 minutes up to a maximum dosage of 3 mg
- verapamil 5 to 10 mg I.V.; may repeat 10 mg after 30 minutes
- procainamide 50 mg/minute by I.V. bolus until the arrhythmia subsides, the QRS complex widens by at least 50%, or the maximum dosage of 1 g has been administered; a continuous infusion of 1 to 4 mg/minute follows.

Nursing implications
- Assess the client for chest pain and rales.
- Provide supplemental oxygen, as prescribed.
- Check the ECG strip to determine what initiated the arrhythmia.
- Have resuscitative equipment available.

POST – TEST 3

ECG characteristics

P wave
Configuration: All normal and alike; one P wave appears for each QRS complex
Rate: 100 beats/minute
Rhythm: Regular

P-R interval 0.22 second

QRS complex
Configuration: All normal and alike
Rate: 100 beats/minute
Rhythm: Regular
Duration: 0.08 second

Interpretation First-degree AV block

Treatment No treatment is needed because the ventricular rate is normal.

Nursing implications
- Monitor the client's serum digoxin level, if indicated.
- Assess the client for more severe degrees of AV block.

POST – TEST 4

ECG characteristics

P wave
Configuration: None
Rate: None
Rhythm: None

P-R interval None

QRS complex	*Configuration:* One wide QRS complex *Rate:* None *Rhythm:* None *Duration:* 0.16 second
Interpretation	Asystole with one agonal beat
Treatment	Begin cardiopulmonary resuscitation. Administer atropine 1 mg I.V. and repeat the dose after 5 minutes. Administer epinephrine 0.5 to 1 mg every 5 minutes. Prepare for temporary pacemaker insertion or defibrillation.
Nursing implications	Monitor the client in more than one lead to rule out fine ventricular fibrillation.

POST – TEST 5

ECG characteristics *P wave*	*Configuration:* None *Rate:* None *Rhythm:* None
P-R interval	None
QRS complex	*Configuration:* Wavy baseline *Rate:* Rapid; cannot be determined precisely *Rhythm:* Irregular *Duration:* None
Interpretation	Ventricular fibrillation
Treatment	Administer a precordial thump if you witness the episode. Defibrillate the client at 200 watts/second and increase to 300 then 360 watts/second if the initial attempt is unsuccessful. Perform cardiopulmonary resuscitation between defibrillation attempts. Administer epinephrine 0.5 to 1 mg I.V. every 5 minutes followed by defibrillation at 360 watts/second. Administer lidocaine 1 mg/kg I.V. followed by 0.5 mg/kg every 5 minutes to a maximum dosage of 3 mg; a continuous infusion of 2 to 4 mg/minute follows. If lidocaine is unsuccessful, administer bretylium 5 to 10 mg/kg followed by continuous infusion at 1 to 2 mg/minute.
Nursing implications	• Prompt recognition and treatment of ventricular fibrillation is a key to successful therapy. • Use a manual resuscitation bag with 100% oxygen to support the client's airway during defibrillation.

POST – TEST 6

ECG characteristics

P wave *Configuration:* Sawtooth flutter waves; the ratio of P waves to QRS complexes is 2:1
Rate: 300 beats/minute
Rhythm: Regular

P-R interval Not measurable

QRS complex *Configuration:* Normal and alike but distorted by the flutter waves
Rate: 150 beats/minute
Rhythm: Regular
Duration: Difficult to measure because of the distortion

Interpretation Atrial flutter

Treatment Synchronized cardioversion at 50 to 100 watts/second is indicated. Pharmacologic therapy may include:
• digoxin 0.25 mg I.V. or by mouth every 6 hours for four doses as a loading dose, then 0.25 mg daily
• quinidine sulfate 200 mg by mouth or intramuscularly every 3 to 4 hours or quinidine gluconate 324 mg every 6 to 8 hours (administer only after digoxin has been started)
• propranolol 10 to 40 mg by mouth four times daily or 1 mg I.V. every 5 minutes up to a maximum dosage of 3 mg
• verapamil 80 mg by mouth three times daily or 5 to 10 mg I.V.; may repeat 10 mg I.V. after 30 minutes
• procainamide 50 mg/minute by I.V. bolus until the arrhythmia subsides, the QRS complex widens by at least 50%, or the maximum initial dosage of 1 g has been administered; a continuous infusion of 1 to 4 mg follows. The oral dose is 250 to 500 mg every 3 hours; that of the slow-release form (Procan SR), 500 mg to 1 g every 6 hours.

Nursing implications • Provide supplemental oxygen, as prescribed.
• Teach the client about cardioversion before the procedure, and obtain an informed consent if time and the client's condition permit.
• Have resuscitative equipment at the client's bedside during cardioversion.

POST – TEST 7

ECG characteristics

P wave *Configuration:* All normal and alike except for the 4th P wave, which is superimposed on the preceding T wave; one P wave appears for each QRS complex
Rate: 75 beats/minute
Rhythm: Regular except for the 4th beat, which is premature

P-R interval 0.18 second

QRS complex *Configuration:* All alike and slightly wide; the 4th QRS complex is slightly different
Rate: 75 beats/minute
Rhythm: Regular except for the 4th beat, which is premature
Duration: 0.12 second

Interpretation Normal sinus rhythm with one premature atrial contraction (PAC)

Treatment No treatment is needed. If PACs become more frequent and are not caused by digoxin toxicity, administer digoxin or quinidine.

Nursing implications
- Explain to the client how caffeine, alcohol, and stress can contribute to PACs. Recommend limited or restricted caffeine and alcohol intake, and teach stress-reduction techniques.
- Monitor the client's serum potassium and digoxin levels; withhold digoxin if serum levels are elevated.
- Observe the ECG monitor for increased frequency of PACs, which may signal the onset of more severe atrial arrhythmias.

POST – TEST 8

ECG characteristics

P wave *Configuration:* None
Rate: Cannot be determined
Rhythm: Cannot be determined

P-R interval None

QRS complex *Configuration:* Wide and bizarre
Rate: About 30 beats/minute
Rhythm: Regular
Duration: 0.14 second

Interpretation   Idioventricular rhythm

Treatment   Administer atropine 0.5 mg I.V. every 5 minutes to a maximum dosage of 2 mg. Prepare for temporary pacemaker insertion. After the maximum dosage of atropine has been administered and until a pacemaker is inserted, administer isoproterenol 2 to 10 mcg/minute.

Nursing implications
- Monitor the serum digoxin and potassium levels.
- Check the hospital's policy for standing orders for administration of atropine.
- Discontinue any lidocaine infusions.

POST – TEST 9

ECG characteristics

P wave   Configuration: All normal and alike; one P wave is not followed by a QRS complex
Rate: 69 beats/minute
Rhythm: Regular

P-R interval   Lengthens progressively from 0.16 to 0.32 second

QRS complex   Configuration: All normal and alike
Rate: About 60 beats/minute
Rhythm: Irregular
Duration: 0.06 second

Interpretation   Second-degree AV block, Mobitz type I

Treatment   No treatment is needed because the ventricular rate is within normal limits. If the ventricular rate decreases and symptoms develop, administer atropine 0.5 mg I.V. every 5 minutes to a maximum dosage of 2 mg. If the bradycardia persists, a temporary pacemaker may be necessary. After the maximum atropine dosage has been administered and until a pacemaker is inserted, administer isoproterenol 2 to 10 mcg/minute.

Nursing implications
- Prepare for possible pacemaker insertion.
- Monitor the client's serum digoxin level.
- Administer supplemental oxygen, as prescribed.

POST – TEST 10

ECG characteristics

P wave   *Configuration:* Normal and alike when visible; one P wave appears for each normal QRS complex
Rate: 130 beats/minute
Rhythm: Regular except when premature beats occur

P-R interval   0.18 second

QRS complex   *Configuration:* Sinus beats are normal and alike; three QRS complexes are wide and bizarre
Rate: 130 beats/minute
Rhythm: Regular except when premature beats occur
Duration: 0.06 second for normal beats; 0.34 second for abnormal beats

Interpretation   Sinus tachycardia with frequent premature ventricular contractions and one episode of ventricular bigeminy

Treatment   Pharmacologic therapy may include:
- lidocaine 1 mg/kg I.V. followed by 0.5 mg/kg every 5 minutes up to a maximum dosage of 3 mg; a continuous infusion of 2 to 4 mg/minute follows
- procainamide 50 mg/minute I.V. until a maximum dosage of 1 g has been administered, the arrhythmia subsides, or the QRS complex widens by at least 50%; a continuous infusion of 1 to 4 mg/minute follows (procainamide is administered if lidocaine proves ineffective)
- bretylium 5 to 10 mg/kg followed by a continuous infusion of 1 to 2 mg/minute (bretylium is administered if lidocaine and procainamide prove ineffective).

Nursing implications
- Check the hospital's policy for standing orders for administration of lidocaine.
- Monitor the client's serum digoxin and potassium levels and arterial blood gas values.
- Administer supplemental oxygen as prescribed.
- Place the client on a cardiac monitor and use an infusion pump when administering antiarrhythmic medications.

POST – TEST 11

ECG characteristics

P wave   *Configuration:* One P wave appears after each QRS complex

Rate: 110 beats/minute
Rhythm: Regular

P-R interval Not measurable

QRS complex *Configuration:* All normal and alike
Rate: 110 beats/minute
Rhythm: Regular
Duration: 0.08 second

Interpretation Junctional tachycardia

Treatment No treatment is needed because the rate is within normal limits.

Nursing implications Monitor the client's serum digoxin level; withhold digoxin if serum levels are elevated.

POST – TEST 12

ECG characteristics
P wave *Configuration:* Normal and alike; P waves march through the QRS complexes
Rate: Not measurable
Rhythm: Not measurable

P-R interval No identifiable pattern emerges

QRS complex *Configuration:* Wide and alike
Rate: Approximately 40 beats/minute
Rhythm: Irregular
Duration: 0.14 second

Interpretation Third-degree AV block

Treatment Administer atropine 0.5 mg I.V. every 5 minutes up to a maximum dosage of 2 mg. A temporary pacemaker may be inserted. Administer isoproterenol 2 to 10 mcg/minute after the maximum atropine dosage has been given and until a pacemaker is inserted.

Nursing implications
• Immediately prepare for pacemaker insertion.
• Place the client in a supine position to reverse hypotension.
• Monitor the client's digoxin level, if indicated.
• Administer supplemental oxygen, as prescribed.

POST – TEST 13

ECG characteristics

P wave   *Configuration:* Wavy baseline
Rate: Not measurable
Rhythm: Irregular

P-R interval   Not measurable

QRS complex   *Configuration:* Normal and alike
Rate: About 130 beats/minute
Rhythm: Irregular
Duration: 0.06 second

Interpretation   Atrial fibrillation

Treatment   Pharmacologic therapy may include:
- digoxin 0.25 mg by mouth daily
- quinidine sulfate 200 mg by mouth every 3 to 4 hours or quinidine gluconate 324 mg by mouth every 6 to 8 hours
- procainamide 250 to 500 mg by mouth every 3 hours; the oral dose of the slow-release form (Procan SR) is 500 mg to 1 g every 6 hours
- propranolol 10 to 40 mg by mouth four times daily
- verapamil 80 mg by mouth three times daily.

Nursing implications
- Assess the client for signs of congestive heart failure, such as rales, dyspnea, and an S_3 gallop.
- Monitor the client's serum digoxin and potassium levels.

POST – TEST 14

ECG characteristics

P wave   *Configuration:* All upright, normal, and alike
Rate: About 47 beats/minute
Rhythm: Regular

P-R interval   0.16 second

QRS complex   *Configuration:* Normal and alike
Rate: About 47 beats/minute
Rhythm: Regular
Duration: 0.08 second

Interpretation   Sinus bradycardia

Treatment If the client develops syncope or hypotension, administer atropine 0.5 mg I.V. every 5 minutes to a maximum dosage of 2 mg. If symptoms persist, administer isoproterenol 2 to 10 mcg/minute until a temporary pacemaker is inserted.

Nursing implications
• Observe the client for signs and symptoms of decreased cardiac output, such as hypotension and decreased level of consciousness.
• Monitor the client's serum digoxin level.

POST – TEST 15

ECG characteristics

P wave *Configuration:* Two normal and alike P waves are visible at the beginning of the strip
Rate: 120 beats/minute
Rhythm: Cannot be determined

P-R interval 0.14 second

QRS complex *Configuration:* The first two QRS complexes are normal and alike; others are wide and bizarre
Rate: 120 beats/minute, then 270 beats/minute
Rhythm: Cannot determine the regularity of the sinus rhythm; a premature complex (3rd beat) precipitates a regular rhythm.
Duration: Sinus beats are 0.08 second; other beats are 0.16 second.

Interpretation Sinus tachycardia that deteriorates to ventricular tachycardia

Treatment If you witness the episode, administer a precordial thump. If the client is conscious and hemodynamically stable:
• administer lidocaine 1 mg/kg I.V. followed by 0.5 mg/kg every 5 minutes to a maximum dosage of 3 mg; a continuous infusion of 2 to 4 mg/minute follows
• administer procainamide 50 mg/minute I.V. until a maximum dosage of 1 g is reached, the arrhythmia subsides, or the QRS complex widens by at least 50%; a continuous infusion of 1 to 4 mg/minute follows (procainamide is administered if lidocaine proves ineffective)
• administer bretylium 5 to 10 mg/kg I.V. followed by a continuous infusion of 1 to 2 mg/minute (bretylium is administered if lidocaine and procainamide prove ineffective)
• administer synchronized cardioversion at 50 to 100 watts/second and repeat, if necessary, at 200, 200 to 300, and 360 watts/second. Sedate a conscious client before cardioversion.

If the client is unconscious or hemodynamically unstable:
- administer synchronized or unsynchronized cardioversion first, then antiarrhythmic agents.

If the client has no pulse:
- defibrillate at 200 watts/second and increase to 300 then 360 watts/second if the initial attempt is unsuccessful
- perform cardiopulmonary resuscitation between defibrillation attempts
- administer antiarrhythmic drugs and epinephrine 0.5 to 1 mg every 5 minutes followed by defibrillation at the maximum 360 watts/second until the arrhythmia is terminated.

Nursing implications   Assess the client quickly to determine the appropriate treatment.

POST – TEST 16

ECG characteristics
P wave   *Configuration:* None seen; the P wave may be buried in the T wave of the preceding beat
Rate: Not measurable
Rhythm: Not measurable

P-R interval   Not measurable

QRS complex   *Configuration:* All normal and alike
Rate: 240 beats/minute
Rhythm: Regular
Duration: 0.10 second

Interpretation   Supraventricular tachycardia (could be either atrial or junctional tachycardia)

Treatment   Carotid sinus massage, synchronized cardioversion at 50 to 100 watts/second, or overdrive pacing is indicated. Pharmacologic therapy may include:
- digoxin 0.25 to 0.50 mg I.V.
- propranolol 1 mg I.V. every 5 minutes up to a maximum dosage of 3 mg
- verapamil 5 to 10 mg I.V.; may repeat 10 mg after 30 minutes
- procainamide 50 mg/minute by I.V. bolus until the arrhythmia subsides, the QRS complex widens by at least 50%, or the maximum initial dosage of 1 g has been administered; a continuous infusion of 1 to 4 mg follows.

Nursing implications
- Check the ECG strip to determine what initiated the arrhythmia.
- Assess the client for chest pain and rales.

- Provide supplemental oxygen, as prescribed.
- Have resuscitative equipment readily available.

POST – TEST 17

ECG characteristics

P wave
Configuration: All normal, upright, and alike
Rate: 85 beats/minute
Rhythm: Regular

P-R interval
0.16 second

QRS complex
Configuration: All normal and alike
Rate: 85 beats/minute
Rhythm: Regular
Duration: 0.04 second

Interpretation
Normal sinus rhythm

Treatment
None

Nursing implications
Continue to observe and monitor the client.

POST – TEST 18

ECG characteristics

P wave
Configuration: None
Rate: Not measurable
Rhythm: Not measurable

P-R interval
Not measurable

QRS complex
Configuration: All wide and alike
Rate: 40 beats/minute
Rhythm: Regular
Duration: 0.12 second

Interpretation
Idioventricular rhythm

Treatment
If the client develops syncope or hypotension, administer atropine 0.5 mg I.V. every 5 minutes to a maximum dosage of 2 mg. Prepare for temporary pacemaker insertion, if necessary.

Nursing implications
Monitor the client's serum digoxin level; withhold digoxin, if indicated.

POST – TEST 19

ECG characteristics

P wave   *Configuration:* All normal and alike; every other P wave is not associated with a QRS complex
Rate: About 90 beats/minute
Rhythm: Regular

P-R interval   0.24 second

QRS complex   *Configuration:* All normal and alike
Rate: About 46 beats/minute
Rhythm: Regular
Duration: 0.08 second

Interpretation   Second-degree AV block, Mobitz type II, with a 2:1 conduction ratio

Treatment   Administer atropine 0.5 mg I.V. every 5 minutes to a maximum dosage of 2 mg. Prepare for temporary pacemaker insertion. Administer isoproterenol 2 to 10 mcg/minute after the maximum atropine dosage has been given and until a pacemaker is inserted.

Nursing implications
- Immediately prepare for pacemaker insertion.
- Place the client in a supine position to reverse hypotension.
- Monitor the client's serum digoxin level, if indicated.
- Administer supplemental oxygen, as ordered.

POST – TEST 20

ECG characteristics

P wave   *Configuration:* None seen
Rate: None
Rhythm: None

P-R interval   Not measurable

QRS complex   *Configuration:* All normal and alike
Rate: 90 beats/minute
Rhythm: Regular
Duration: 0.08 second

Interpretation   Accelerated junctional rhythm

Treatment   No treatment is needed. Administer atropine if the heart rate decreases and hypotension or syncope develops.

Nursing implications
- Monitor the client's serum digoxin level; withhold digoxin if indicated.
- Consult with the physician about withholding antiarrhythmic medications.

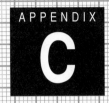

Nursing Care Plans for Selected Arrhythmias

NURSING CARE PLAN FOR A CLIENT WITH:

Sinus Bradycardia
Sinus Arrest or Exit Block
Junctional Rhythm
Atrioventricular Block
Idioventricular Rhythm

Nursing Diagnosis Decreased cardiac output related to low heart rate

Expected Outcomes
- The client maintains hemodynamic stability as evidenced by a heart rate greater than ___ and a blood pressure greater than ___ (specify parameters).
- The client does not experience changes in mental status, such as dizziness or syncope.

Nursing Interventions
- Document episodes of the arrhythmia by obtaining an ECG strip; continue to monitor heart rhythm.
- Assess for changes in blood pressure and peripheral pulse rates.
- Assess for changes in mental status, such as dizziness and syncope.
- Monitor the client's serum digoxin and potassium levels.
- Withhold all medications that slow conduction (for example, digoxin, lidocaine, verapamil).

If hypotension and changes in mental status occur:
- Place the client in a supine position.
- Establish intravenous access, if necessary.
- Administer oxygen, as ordered.
- Confer with the physician if there is no standing order for atropine.
- Administer atropine according to the institution's standing order protocol or the physician's order.
- Evaluate atropine's effectiveness in meeting the expected outcomes.
- Prepare for isoproterenol administration or pacemaker insertion.
- Prepare the client for transfer to the intensive care unit, if necessary.

Nursing Diagnosis Potential for injury related to decreased cerebral blood flow

Expected Outcome The client avoids physical injury during episodes of arrhythmia.

Nursing Interventions
- Assess and document changes in mental status to determine the risk of injury.
- Maintain bed rest and keep side rails up.
- Place the client in a supine position to increase blood flow to the brain.
- Consider using soft restraints if the client becomes restless or agitated.

- Decrease environmental stimuli: discourage visitors and reduce noise and light.
- Stay with the client throughout an arrhythmic episode.
- Reorient the client to the environment, as necessary.

NURSING CARE PLAN FOR A CLIENT WITH:

Sinus Tachycardia
Atrial Fibrillation
Atrial Flutter
Junctional Tachycardia
Atrial Tachycardia

Nursing Diagnosis   Decreased cardiac output related to decreased ventricular filling time

Expected Outcomes
- The client maintains hemodynamic stability as evidenced by a heart rate less than ___ and a blood pressure greater than ___ (specify parameters).
- The client does not experience changes in mental status, such as dizziness or syncope.

Nursing Interventions
- Document episodes of the arrhythmia by obtaining an ECG strip; continue to monitor heart rhythm.
- Assess for changes in blood pressure and peripheral pulse rates; monitor for jugular vein distention.
- Assess for changes in mental status, such as dizziness and syncope.
- For sinus tachycardia:
—Assess for possible causes of arrhythmia: pain, fever, anxiety, hypoxia, and anemia.
—Monitor arterial blood gas, hemoglobin, and hematocrit values.
—Notify the physician of any change in the client's status; administer therapy as ordered.
—Have resuscitative equipment available if the physician performs carotid sinus massage to differentiate sinus tachycardia (carotid sinus massage will temporarily slow sinus tachycardia).
- For atrial fibrillation:
—Monitor the serum potassium level.
—Assess for pulse deficit on apical-radial pulse assessment.
—Prepare for possible synchronized cardioversion.
—Have resuscitative equipment available.
- For atrial flutter:
—Have resuscitative equipment available for possible cardioversion or carotid sinus massage.
- For atrial tachycardia:
—Check the ECG strip for the event triggering the arrhythmia.

—Have resuscitative equipment available for possible cardioversion or carotid sinus massage.
—Monitor the serum digoxin level if atrial tachycardia with block occurs.
• For junctional tachycardia:
—Monitor the ECG strip for the event triggering the arrhythmia.
—Have resuscitative equipment available for possible cardioversion or carotid sinus massage.
—Monitor the serum digoxin level.
—Avoid administering antiarrhythmic medications if the junctional tachycardia is associated with an inferior wall myocardial infarction; antiarrhythmic agents may worsen the arrhythmia.

Nursing Diagnosis   Chest pain related to decreased coronary artery perfusion

Expected Outcomes
• The client is free of chest pain during and after tachyarrhythmia.
• The client expresses relief from chest pain by ___ (specify time).

Nursing Interventions
• Assess and document chest pain:
—Severity: Ask the client to rate pain on a scale of 1 to 10.
—Quality: Ask the client to describe the pain.
—Location: Ask the client to point to where it hurts.
• Assess for objective signs of pain: grimacing, clutching chest, increased blood pressure and respiratory rate, diaphoresis.
• Provide supplemental oxygen, as prescribed.
• Maintain bed rest; provide comfort measures, such as relaxation techniques and positioning.
• Administer nitroglycerin or morphine sulfate, as prescribed; monitor and document the effectiveness of pain medications.

NURSING CARE PLAN FOR A CLIENT WITH:

Asystole

Nursing Diagnosis   Decreased cardiac output related to lack of heart rate and circulation

Expected Outcomes
• The client maintains adequate circulation during the arrhythmia as evidenced by a palpable peripheral pulse during cardiopulmonary resuscitation (CPR).
• The client has a prompt restoration of an adequate heart rhythm, heart rate, and blood pressure.

Nursing Interventions
• Immediately begin CPR.
• Notify the code team according to hospital protocol.

- Monitor the client in more than one lead to rule out ventricular fibrillation.
- Prepare medications for possible infusion: epinephrine, atropine, isoproterenol.
- Prepare for temporary pacing, either transcutaneous or transvenous.
- Monitor the effectiveness of CPR by checking for a palpable peripheral pulse.
- Monitor the client continuously for a change in rhythm; assess pulse rate and blood pressure when the change is noted.

Nursing Diagnosis   Impaired gas exchange related to a lack of circulatory transport of oxygen and carbon dioxide

Expected Outcome   The client maintains adequate ventilation during the arrhythmia as evidenced by symmetrical chest excursion and bilateral breath sounds during manual aeration and by restoration of the client's Pa_{O_2}, Pa_{CO_2}, and pH toward normal ranges.

Nursing Interventions
- Institute appropriate artificial ventilation.
- Make the transition to aeration with 100% oxygen delivered by manual resuscitation bag as soon as possible.
- Prepare for endotracheal intubation.
- Observe for bilateral chest expansion.
- Auscultate for bilateral breath sounds.
- Monitor arterial blood gas values.
- Consult with the physician about a follow-up chest X-ray to confirm endotracheal tube placement.
- Assist with the transition to mechanical ventilation as soon as the arrhythmia is terminated.

NURSING CARE PLAN FOR A CLIENT WITH:

Temporary Pacemaker

Nursing Diagnosis   Decreased cardiac output related to pacemaker malfunction

Expected Outcome   The client maintains a heart rate greater than ___ (specify) and evidence of proper sensing and pacing of pacemaker.

Nursing Interventions
- Record and document any incident of pacemaker malfunction.
- Assess the ECG strip for proper pacing and sensing.
- Check the pulse generator for power and proper milliamperes, heart rate, and sensitivity settings.

- Adjust the milliampere or sensitivity setting according to institutional policy to achieve the desired outcome.
- Ensure proper tightness of all connections from the pulse generator to the catheter.
- Change the battery regularly (according to institutional policy) and whenever the pacemaker malfunctions.
- Reposition the client to attempt to move the catheter back into position.
- Notify the physician of pacemaker malfunction, and prepare for possible catheter manipulation.

Nursing Diagnosis Potential for injury related to microshock

Expected Outcome The client is free of unexplained sustained ventricular arrhythmias while the pacing catheter is in place.

Nursing Interventions
- Place all terminals and the pulse generator in a rubber glove.
- Cover the catheter with insulated tips when it is disconnected from the pulse generator.
- Wear rubber gloves when handling the catheter.
- Avoid using ungrounded electrical equipment near the client.
- Check all electrical equipment for ungrounded prongs and frayed wires.
- Do not touch the client and electrical equipment simultaneously.
- Investigate all electrical equipment when unexplained sustained ventricular arrhythmia occurs.

NURSING CARE PLAN FOR A CLIENT WITH:

Premature Ventricular Contractions
Ventricular Tachycardia with a Pulse

Nursing Diagnosis Decreased cardiac output related to abnormal pumping action of the heart

Expected Outcome The client demonstrates hemodynamic stability as evidenced by restoration of a normal heart rhythm; blood pressure and pulse rate are within normal limits for the client (specify).

Nursing Interventions
- Document and record evidence of the arrhythmia; continuously monitor the client's heart rhythm.
- Monitor the client's blood pressure and level of consciousness.
- Place the client in a supine position if hypotension or decreased level of consciousness develops.
- Know the institution's standing order protocol for lidocaine administration.

- Prepare to administer antiarrhythmic medications; use an infusion pump for continuous administration.
- Notify the physician of the arrhythmia.
- For sustained ventricular tachycardia:
—Administer a precordial thump if you witness the episode.
—Prepare the client for possible cardioversion.
- Have resuscitative equipment available.
- Monitor the client's blood pressure after the arrhythmia is terminated.

Nursing Diagnosis   Impaired gas exchange related to decreased circulatory transport of oxygen and carbon dioxide

Expected Outcome   The client demonstrates adequate ventilation as evidenced by a respiratory rate, PaO_2, $PaCO_2$, and pH within normal limits for the client (specify).

Nursing Interventions
- Assess and document the client's respiratory rate and any evidence of difficulty in breathing.
- Monitor arterial blood gas values.
- Place the client in semi-Fowler's position if not contraindicated by hypotension.
- Administer supplemental oxygen, as prescribed.
- Manually aerate the client with 100% oxygen, if necessary.
- Prepare for possible endotracheal intubation.

NURSING CARE PLAN FOR A CLIENT WITH:

Ventricular Fibrillation
Pulseless Ventricular Tachycardia

Nursing Diagnosis   Decreased cardiac output related to abnormal pumping action of the heart

Expected Outcome   The client demonstrates hemodynamic stability as evidenced by restoration of a normal heart rhythm; blood pressure and pulse rate are within normal limits for the client (specify).

Nursing Interventions
- Administer a precordial thump if you witness the episode.
- Begin CPR.
- Notify the code team.
- Know the institution's standing order protocols for defibrillation and lidocaine administration.

- Immediately defibrillate at 200 watts/second; repeat at 200 to 300 and 360 watts/second, if necessary.
- Prepare medications for possible administration: epinephrine, lidocaine, procainamide, and bretylium.
- Continuously monitor heart rhythm; monitor blood pressure after the arrhythmia is terminated.

Nursing Diagnosis Impaired gas exchange related to lack of circulatory transport of oxygen and carbon dioxide

Expected Outcome The client maintains adequate ventilation during the arrhythmia as evidenced by symmetrical chest excursion and bilateral breath sounds during manual aeration and by restoration of the client's Pa_{O_2}, Pa_{CO_2}, and pH toward normal ranges.

Nursing Interventions
- Institute appropriate artificial ventilation.
- Make the transition to aeration with 100% oxygen delivered by manual resuscitation bag as soon as possible.
- Prepare for endotracheal intubation.
- Observe for bilateral chest expansion.
- Auscultate for bilateral breath sounds.
- Monitor arterial blood gas values.
- Consult with the physician about a follow-up chest X-ray to confirm endotracheal tube placement.
- Assist with the transition to mechanical ventilation when the arrhythmia is terminated.

INDIVIDUALIZING CLIENT CARE

Use the form on the opposite page to individualize client care.

NURSING CARE PLAN FOR A CLIENT WITH:

_____

_____

Nursing Diagnosis   _____

_____

_____

_____

_____

_____

Expected Outcome   _____

_____

_____

_____

_____

_____

Nursing Interventions   _____

_____

_____

_____

_____

_____

_____

_____

_____

_____

_____

Selected References

Conover, M. *Pocket Nurse Guide to Electrocardiography.* St. Louis: C.V. Mosby Co., 1986.

Conover, M. *Understanding Electrocardiography: Arrhythmias and the 12-Lead ECG,* 5th ed. St. Louis: C.V. Mosby Co., 1988.

Davis, D. *How to Quickly and Accurately Master ECG Interpretation.* Philadelphia: J.B. Lippincott, 1985.

EKG Cards. Springhouse, Pa.: Springhouse Corp., 1987.

Fassler, M., and Steuble, B. *Electrocardiogram Interpretation and Emergency Intervention.* Springhouse, Pa.: Springhouse Corp., 1991.

Horvath, P.T. *Care of the Adult Cardiac Surgery Patient.* New York: John Wiley & Sons, 1984.

Huszar, R.J. *Basic Dysrhythmias: Interpretation and Management.* St. Louis: C.V. Mosby Co., 1988.

Johnson, R., and Schwartz, M.H. *A Simplified Approach to Electrocardiography.* Philadelphia: W.B. Saunders, 1986.

Krasover, T. "A Conceptual Approach to the Electrocardiogram," *Critical Care Nurse* 66-76, March/April 1982.

Marriott, H.J.L. *Practical Electrocardiography,* 8th ed. Baltimore: Williams & Wilkins, 1988.

Weller, D., and Noone, J. "Mechanisms of Arrhythmia: Enhanced Automaticity and Reentry," *Critical Care Nurse* 42-66, May 1989.

Index

i refers to an illustration; t, to a table.

i refers to an illustration; t, to a table.